Bion's Transformations Revisited and Expanded

In this illuminating volume, Arnaldo Chuster provides a thorough critique of Wilfred Bion's seminal 1965 work, *Transformations*.

Offering a rich and nuanced opportunity to enhance one's understanding of this pivotal psychoanalytic text, Chuster establishes a link between the practice of psychoanalysis and Bion's advanced theory, including the key challenges he encountered in the clinical setting with patients. Working through *Transformations*, Chuster embarks on a courageous journey to follow Bion's path in creating a dialogue between multiple disciplines, explicating and expanding upon the core concepts of different types of transformation. Chuster recognizes *Transformations* as a pivotal point in Bion's publications, highlighting the profound manifestations of complex thinking it exhibits. Following the complexities of Bion's ideas, the book offers invaluable insights and expansions on topics such as ethics, aesthetics, and their application in imaginative conjectures, while also providing a rigorous discussion on the scientific foundations of Bion's work.

Chuster's innovative perspectives and dedication to the work of Bion make this book a must-read for all psychoanalysts interested in demystifying the often convoluted work of this most eminent analyst and bringing his insightful theories into the 21st century.

Arnaldo Chuster is a Training and Supervising Analyst at the Rio de Janeiro Psychoanalytic Society (SPRJ), affiliated with the International Psychoanalytic Association (IPA), as well as a member of the Newport Psychoanalytic Institute (NPI) in California, and an honorary member and Professor at the W.R. Bion Institute, Porto Alegre, Brazil.

Elahe Sagart is a psychiatrist and psychoanalyst with a private practice in Newport Beach, California. She specializes in Child, Adolescent, and Adult Psychoanalysis and serves as a core faculty member at the New Center for Psychoanalysis (NCP) in Los Angeles, CA. Dr. Sagart is a member of both the International Psychoanalytical Association (IPA) and the American Psychoanalytic Association (APsaA). She is also the founder of the Rustin Psychoanalytic Group in Tehran, Iran.

The Routledge Wilfred R. Bion Studies Book Series

Series Editor

Howard B. Levine, MD

The contributions of Wilfred Bion are among the most cited in the analytic literature. Their appeal lies not only in their content and explanatory value, but in their generative potential. Although Bion's training and many of his clinical instincts were deeply rooted in the classical tradition of Melanie Klein, his ideas have a potentially universal appeal. Rather than emphasizing a particular psychic content (e.g., Oedipal conflicts in need of resolution; splits that needed to be healed; preconceived transferences that must be allowed to form and flourish, etc.), he tried to help open and prepare the mind of the analyst (without memory, desire or theoretical preconception) for the encounter with the patient.

Bion's formulations of group mentality and the psychotic and non-psychotic portions of the mind, his theory of thinking and emphasis on facing and articulating the truth of one's existence so that one might truly learn firsthand from one's own experience, his description of psychic development (alpha function and container/contained) and his exploration of **O** are "non-denominational" concepts that defy relegation to a particular school or orientation of psychoanalysis. Consequently, his ideas have taken root in many places.... and those ideas continue to inform many different branches of psychoanalytic inquiry and interest.[1]

It is with this heritage and its promise for the future developments of psychoanalysis in mind that we present *The Routledge Wilfred Bion Studies Book Series*. This series gathers together newly emerging and continually evolving contributions to psychoanalytic thinking that rest upon Bion's foundational texts and explore and extend the implications of his thought.

Note

1 H.B. Levine and G. Civitarese. Editors' Preface, *The W.R. Bion Tradition*, Levine and Civitarese, eds., 2016, Karnac, p. xxi.

For a full list of titles in the series, please visit the Routledge website at: https://www.routledge.com/The-Routledge-Wilfred-Bion-Studies-Book-Series/book-series/RWBSBS

Bion's Transformations Revisited and Expanded

Essays on the Complexity of Psychoanalysis

Arnaldo Chuster

Edited by Elahe Sagart

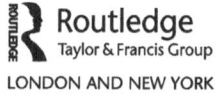

Routledge
Taylor & Francis Group

LONDON AND NEW YORK

Designed cover image: Photo by Behzad Bernous, Psy.D.

First published 2025
by Routledge
4 Park Square, Milton Park, Abingdon, Oxon OX14 4RN

and by Routledge
605 Third Avenue, New York, NY 10158

*Routledge is an imprint of the Taylor & Francis Group, an informa
business*

© 2025 Arnaldo Chuster

British Library Cataloguing-in-Publication Data
A catalogue record for this book is available from the British Library

ISBN: 978-1-032-75466-6 (hbk)
ISBN: 978-1-032-74806-1 (pbk)
ISBN: 978-1-003-47412-8 (ebk)

DOI: 10.4324/9781003474128

Typeset in Times New Roman
by KnowledgeWorks Global Ltd.

Contents

Acknowledgements

I am delighted to express my heartfelt gratitude to Elahe Sagart for her generous assistance and insightful critiques throughout the meticulous review and editing process of this book. Her contributions have been invaluable, and without her support, the task of bringing this publication to fruition would have been nearly impossible.

My gratitude extends to several colleagues for their support and insightful critiques during our Bion study group meetings since 2002. Special appreciation goes to James Ogilvie, Afsaneh Alisobhani, Glenda Corstorphine, Kirby Ogden, Karen Willette, Thomas Helscher, Robin Goldberg, Jeffrey Eaton, Marianne Robinson, Shirley Gooch, James Gooch, and Avner Bernstein for their constructive feedback.

Special acknowledgment is conveyed to the study group on Bion's ideas, composed of Elahe Sagart, Mark Santarelli, Rachel Bartur, Carol Hekman, and Marina Ribeiro. In addition, special thanks are extended to the former participants Mara Thorsen, Glenn Mowbray, Chao-Ying Wang, Judith Goodman, Janet Smith, and Joshua Richmond.

Furthermore, I am grateful to Howard Levine for his dedicated efforts and support in the publication process.

In special tribute, I express my deepest gratitude to the memories of James Grotstein and James Gooch. Their generosity to explore and affirm my wild thoughts has left a lasting impression, and their encouragement is profoundly valued.

Arnaldo Chuster, M.D.

Editor's Preface

I first met Arnaldo Chuster in Pasadena, CA, in 2014, during a lecture on Bion's work organized by the Newport Psychoanalytic Institute. I was fortunate to attend this lecture, thanks to an invitation from my friend Afsaneh Alisobhani. At the time, Chuster's new book, *Lonesome Road: Essays on the Complexity of W.R. Bion's Work*, had just been released. My familiarity with his work began through James Gooch, a Los Angeles-based Bion scholar, who was keenly interested in Chuster's insights on Bion's concepts.

Navigating through disciplines is invariably challenging, more so when diving into Bion's most intricate work, *Transformations*. Chuster embarks on a bold expedition, tracing Bion's footsteps to foster a dialogue across multiple disciplines. He skillfully elucidates and expands upon the fundamental concepts of various transformations. Chuster's vast expertise spans diverse subjects, from philosophy and mythology to mathematics, among others. This extensive knowledge marks him as a faithful follower of Bion, adept at weaving psychoanalysis with other domains at a conceptual level.

Chuster's contributions go beyond theoretical discourse, offering an enriching learning experience that links psychoanalytic practice with the core theories within a Bionian framework. Sharing challenging clinical encounters, he provides nuanced insights into these complex interactions. Chuster's innovative approach not only sparks profound curiosity but also leads readers on an intense journey through the depths of Bion's seminal book, "Transformations." His dedication and passion for Bion's work and psychoanalysis command respect and admiration.

In conclusion, I wish to emphasize several aspects of this book and its approach. This work is not intended as an introductory guide to Bion's theories; rather, it assumes a significant familiarity with Bion's foundational concepts on the part of the reader. The reader will notice a focused reference to psychoanalytic literature, including the work of other Bion scholars. This approach is due to the book's foundation on Chuster's interpretation of Bion's theories, leading to frequent citations of his own previously published works. Furthermore, the text revisits certain themes to underscore their inherent interconnections and deepen understanding through various analytical perspectives.

Reflecting on my role in this project, I am grateful for Chuster's confidence in entrusting me with the editing of his book and appreciate his patience through the meticulous revisions and his assistance in clarifying complex concepts. Despite my lack of prior editing experience, with this being my inaugural project, I regard this undertaking as a profound learning opportunity, embodying the principle of Learning from Experience. It indeed challenged my resilience and proved to be a transformative journey for me. I kindly ask the reader to gracefully forgive any editorial shortcomings. It is my sincere hope that this book brings as much joy and insight to its readers as it has to me throughout the editing process.

Elahe Sagart, M.D.

Introduction

I

It is widely acknowledged that psychoanalysis produced remarkable transformations in human knowledge through its irreplaceable observations of the *unconscious* roots inherent in all human realizations. These observations profoundly influenced *aesthetics*, a phenomenon explicitly recognized by Freud himself in 1926, and introduced a new way of conceptualizing the *ethics of thinking*.

This novel approach to ethics and aesthetics created a distinctive practice in human history, centering on the alleviation of psychic pain and its broader implications in life. Consequently, it became inevitable to delve into intricate topics such as emotional experiences, choices in life, perceptions of time, maturity, social autonomy, responsibility, and the nuanced associations inherent in the broad meanings of these terms.

Navigating this complex landscape confronts a psychoanalyst with multifaceted experiences, necessitating prudent decisions regarding inclusion or exclusion. This may pertain to oneself within diverse groups, a patient within one's practice, or the incorporation or omission of interpretations, associations, ideas, and theories. Mastery in managing these complexities is anchored in a comprehensive understanding of psychoanalytic practice and its perpetual transformations.

Having devoted nearly five decades to the study and teaching of psychoanalysis, and perceiving psychoanalysis as a science predicated on the observation of human connections through the unconscious vertex, I encountered a complementary perspective by Castoriadis (1997): psychoanalysis is a "*practical-poietic activity*." From my standpoint, this definition is dynamic, encapsulating both ethical and aesthetic dimensions, and aligns seamlessly with Bion's theoretical developments, akin to a perfectly tailored glove.

This definition highlights the importance Bion attributed to achieving a mental state akin to that of poets and artists, albeit with a cautionary note to psychoanalysts regarding the demands of embodying a poet or artist. Yet, there exists a profound historical juncture, an *idée mère*,[1] where distinguishing between these activities becomes challenging, if not impossible.

DOI: 10.4324/9781003474128-1

I advocate for the application of an *undecidability principle of origin*[2] that weaves together science, poetry, philosophy, and psychoanalysis. I designate the term "*poietic threshold*" to signify a critical juncture where psychoanalytic language can flourish, drawing sustenance from evolving notions of aesthetics and ethics.

In Bion's writings, this poietic threshold consistently emerges at the core of practical activity. This activity, extending beyond the alleviation of psychic pain, heralds a singular paradigm in human history with the capacity to enhance, ameliorate, and, fundamentally, safeguard human thought, thereby elevating the quality of psychic life.

Engaging with this threshold entails wrestling with complexity. Hence, in the present volume, I endeavor to examine how Bion's theories offer sanctuary for human thought through a *psychoanalytic Theory of Complexity*.[3]

I regard Bion as the pioneering intellect who introduced the vertex of complexity within the domain of psychoanalysis. Acknowledging his seminal contributions in *Transformations* (Bion, 1965) and its subsequent developments as both profound and exemplary, I am compelled to dedicate the present volume to a thorough examination of this theme.

II

Bion, with intuitive foresight, applied the principles of complexity theory to psychoanalysis, despite being ostensibly unfamiliar with the formal theory at the time. His extensive consultations across mathematics, epistemology, philosophy, and the forefronts of modern science likely steered his intuitively gifted mind toward such a direction. Viewing *Transformations* (1965) as a particularly challenging segment of Bion's work, I contend that appreciating the complexity vertex renders its intricate concepts distinctly comprehensible. Consequently, a primary task in this book is to embrace this challenge head-on, employing and highlighting tools from the theory of complexity embedded within Bion's propositions.

Bion's application of the theory of complexity to psychoanalysis, as vividly unfolded in his book *Transformations*, may explain why, over the years, his writings simultaneously infuriated and captivated his readers. He inspired a broad spectrum of emotions, ranging from curiosity to despair, reverence to disdain, and perplexity to awe. The diversity of dense topics Bion addressed, through innovative ideas and a novel stylistic approach, inevitably polarized opinions. For an extended period, across numerous psychoanalytic institutes, his works were paradoxically revered and censured, at times excluded from the recommended readings list. Yet, both proponents and critics attest to his unwavering ethical integrity and profound respect for others.

Bion was a visionary, projecting himself into the future with his robust intuition coupled with an extensive capacity to inquire and elucidate the pressing questions of his era—and it would be a disservice to confine his relevance to "*his time*" alone. Even in contemporary discourse, Bion's far-reaching ideas continue to surpass temporal boundaries.

III

Philosophers of science dedicate special attention to the essence of scientific revolutions, recognizing that each revolution is ushered in by geniuses—individuals whose remarkable capacities and, most notably, their powerful imagination, compel the scientific community to abandon old thinking habits in favor of novel and uncharted concepts. In the trajectory of scientific advancement, shifts in methodologies profoundly impact the emergence of innovations and ideas. In this context, Bion emerged as an analyst who fundamentally altered the path of psychoanalytic discourse not only by the introduction of new ideas but also by reshaping the very method of psychoanalytic inquiry. His distinctive style, marked by a blend of humorous respect and sharp critique of the knowledge acquired through psychoanalysis, sets him apart.

In an idiosyncratic manner, Bion demonstrated a singular talent for re-approaching numerous traditional psychoanalytic themes, such as free-floating attention, resistance, the Oedipus complex, the language of interpretation, settings, and ethics, from fresh vantage points. He discarded the characteristic formalism of classical psychoanalysis and developed a creative, yet intuitive, methodology for psychoanalytic practice. His style encourages us to abandon rigid formalism in favor of an authentic engagement in the analytic encounter, particularly in the articulation of our thoughts and ideas. Nevertheless, embracing this style is extremely challenging, necessitating an inward tap into the genius within us, potentially directing our curiosity almost exclusively at daunting questions (Chuster 1989, 2014, 2018a).

IV

Bion's distinctive life experiences and his ever-expanding mind presented him with a series of intriguing challenges and puzzles. This exposure empowered him to fearlessly confront the technical complexities inherent in psychoanalysis.

From the outset of his practice, Bion placed a special emphasis on observing the *ever-changing* subject, which required the integration of different vertices and disciplines. This innovative approach demanded patience in unraveling mysteries by generating new links while avoiding premature conclusions. In 1970, Bion encapsulated this proposition by adopting Keats's notion of *negative capability* (1817)— the poet's exceptional ability, "which Shakespeare possessed so enormously," to embrace "uncertainties, mysteries, doubts, without any irritable reaching after fact and reason." An evident outcome of this capacity is reflected in Bion's theory of thinking (1962a), which integrates the complexity of dialogue across various disciplines, including psychoanalysis, philosophy, pure mathematics, and applied mathematics (Chuster, 2014, 2018, 2018a).

It is crucial to note that Bion did not directly engage with mathematics or philosophy per se. Instead, he created a network in search of new inquiries relevant to psychoanalysis, or at the very least, proposing a novel way to articulate them. This endeavor involved multiple vertices, aiming for a more ambitious goal in *Transformations* (1965), wherein the dialogue among psychoanalysis, art, and mathematics sought to achieve for psychoanalysis what non-Euclidean space did for geometry. This bold move encountered significant institutional opposition and resulted in the withdrawal of some readers.

Another objective in this book, as I review Bion's propositions in *Transformations* (1965), is to examine the interconnection between aesthetics, ethics, psychoanalysis, and mathematics as an exemplification of Complexity. My aim is to demonstrate that the primary instrument for understanding Bion's ideas, alongside applying the Theory of Complexity, relies on an additional critical element: the depth of our imaginative capacity in psychoanalytic thought.

V

The popular concept of complexity has always been present in daily vocabulary, often signifying something confusing, difficult to understand, or relating to objects with numerous interconnected elements. Edgar Morin was the first thinker to expand on the scientific vertex of complexity.[4]

Morin built upon the revolution sparked by Austrian mathematician Kurt Gödel's[5] theorems, which led to a significant epistemological shift in *axiomatic systems*. These theorems laid the groundwork for conceptualizing so-called *open systems*, markedly altering scientific and philosophical thought to embrace a new paradigm. Thanks to Bion, a paradigmatic shift is seamlessly integrated into psychoanalytic thinking and practice.

In essence, the primary reason for adopting a complexity framework is to challenge our natural inclination toward *closed systems,* grounded in classification and simple computation. Such systems frequently adopt a diagnostic approach in clinical practice, potentially obstructing the acceptance of novel ideas. In contrast, complexity embraces open interactions and qualities that defy the conventional rules of calculation. It encompasses uncertainties, random phenomena, chaos, and a significant dialogue between chance and choice.

Moreover, complexity can be linked to the most important emotional experiences that contribute to the development of the mind, particularly those of a *passionate nature*, where love, hatred, and the thirst for the truth are integrated rather than split into separate objects. This represents a shift in the method and logic of emotional experience, essentially connecting open systems to the work of our imagination and allowing the experience of *wild thoughts*[6] to enrich or even provide meaning to mental life.

This book attempts to share some of my "wild thoughts" through the vertex of complexity. In doing so, a space is opened for discussing concepts such as the spectrum model of the psychotic/non-psychotic parts of the personality, the theory of thinking, the psychoanalytic object, the Grid, "O," transformations as a theory of catastrophe, transformations in "O," thoughts without a thinker, emotional turbulence, the act of faith, at-one-ment, negative capability, and the language of achievement.

Bion's intricate thought process has established a bridge between different disciplines, carving out a new psychoanalytic space that defies exclusive alignment with any single domain. This bridge facilitates the flow of imaginative and wild thoughts, confronting scientific knots, venturing into the uncertainty of ideas, and grappling with contradictions in logic. The overarching goal is to engender a perpetual state of tension in the pursuit of knowledge (K link).

It is essential to recognize that the K link aligns with the incompleteness of psychoanalytic investigation. This incompleteness also signifies the impossibility of obtaining answers to the major dilemmas that plague humanity. Nevertheless, it fosters a *dialogic perspective*, a Heraclitean vertex that views the world as an eternal battlefield for navigating the challenges of existence amidst diverse logics.

Complexity demands the endurance of paradoxes and contradictions for as long as necessary. Meanwhile, we ought to leverage our imagination to forge meaning or, at the very least, to foresee the potential awakenings within us, paving the way for discoveries across a spectrum of transformations.

I have attempted to discuss such a spectrum in various papers, employing an epistemological instrument named the *ethical-aesthetical principles* (Chuster, 1999, 2002, 2014, 2018). In this book, they are inevitably referenced in numerous sections. Furthermore, it is imperative to engage with many ideas presented in the works *Attention and Interpretation* (1970), *The Grid and Caesura* (1977), and the so-called *Four Papers*, as they naturally evolve from *Transformations* (1965).

VI

Bion's model of *pre-conception, searching for a realization and giving birth to a conception,* when viewed through the lens of the ethical-aesthetical principles of complexity, offers a novel trajectory for understanding human evolution. This approach is indeed a portrayal of the complexity Bion referred to as "O" (1965).

The pre-conception model aligns closely with the genetics theory that humans are *neotenic* beings, suggesting that human infants are born in a state of profound immaturity. This evolutionary strategy, reducing innate predispositions to enhance the capacity for experiential learning, served as a survival mechanism in a perilous world (Chuster, 2014, 2018b). This is a significant theoretical discussion in psychoanalysis, as the traditional Freudian model of drives provides an approximation in understanding the crucial limits between the body and mind. Bion's neotenic human is not just a fictional approach but a translation of human genetic development over time. It illustrates how humans have managed to survive by transforming reality to acknowledge the existence of the mind, even though humanity has yet to properly address cruelty and destruction.

Human existence is deeply entwined with *learning from emotional experiences* and the ability to locate such experiences within the enigmatic realm of mind. Descriptions of failures in this process have extensively been explored throughout Bion's work.

The inherent complexity of the pre-conception model has two products: the domain of thoughts and language. This encompasses the creation of meanings and words, and their impact on the interaction between the physical and the social body, necessitating a multidimensional field for understanding.

Every *thought* (*conceptions and concepts*) denotes an *indeterminate* state, a reality forever open to transformations, constituted through a fundamental link where the container and the contained incessantly interact within the limits of the *alpha function's capacity*—an extension of the interaction of the mother-infant dyad, which forms the basic link of the *reverie function*. Their distinction is clear: reverie is primarily (though not exclusively) sensorial, while the alpha function is mainly symbolic (though not exclusively). Note that the spectrum model offers a more complex and sophisticated perspective than Freud's delineation of the boundary between body and mind, enhancing our understanding of his model of drives and structures.

This essential foundational link is pivotal to the analytic process, manifesting as *indeterminacy* in psychoanalysis through transformations of the associative process. For instance, the trajectory of a patient's associations following a dream recount or the unpredictable shifts in mental states post-interpretation exemplify the ethical-aesthetical principles of Uncertainty and its corollary, the principle of Incompleteness.

Another outcome of this link is its infinite nature, which I (1999, 2002, 2014, and 2018) identified as the *principle of infinity*. This suggests that the human unconscious extends far beyond the conventional Freudian Unconscious. Discussing the Unconscious already places one outside the subject, indicating an expanded unconscious that necessitates fresh interpretation. Occasionally, it becomes necessary to introduce a new term to the discourse, with "*inaccessible*" being the closest term for Bion, embodying another ethical-aesthetical principle through an *undecidability principle*.

Austrian mathematician Kurt Gödel was the first to articulate this principle, later becoming foundational for Heisenberg's Uncertainty principle. The *undecidability principle* asserts that within every living link, there exists a point of ambiguity regarding its ownership.

The most crucial pre-conception for psychoanalysis is the Oedipal preconception, as it includes all others (Chuster, 2002, 2014, 2018, 2022). Once again, applying the principle of complexity suggests that we should think beyond the classical application of the theory of the Oedipus complex.

For instance, when the analyst draws associations with the myth of Oedipus, these associations will invariably differ at various moments in their practice, and their outcomes remain unpredictable. Another significant characteristic of oedipal preconceptions is their continual reducibility to the mental world. For instance, the infant initially seeks the mother's mind to reach the physical breast, not the contrary. Therefore, a triangle is formed: the mind of the infant, the mind of the mother, and the breast.

Within this tridimensional space, the mother's mind reserves a place to receive the infant's pre-conception, whereupon a conception emerges between them. In this creative space, the infant perceives the rhythm of the milk flow, the gentleness of the mother's love, and the emotional warmth that arises in a secure environment. This model elucidates why some children struggle to take the breast when the mother's mind is absent or why individuals may dissociate between the material and psychic breast when the mother is distracted from the infant (Bion, 1962a).

In a complementary and *autopoietic looping* manner, the Oedipal preconception seeks the minds of the parents to mate with the reality of the family, just as the family seeks to connect with society, and society seeks creations to support various levels of nurturing infants. If this integration occurs inadequately, an individual may spend their life in a state of feeling pain with no suffering, indicating an inability to solve problems due to their incapacity to confront them.

The realizations of the Oedipal pre-conception unfold across a spectrum of possibilities for conceptions and concepts. Being a non-structural model, it presents many challenges for those unfamiliar with it.

At one end of the spectrum is *social-ism*, opposed to *narcissism* at the other. This spectrum represents one facet of the *psychoanalytic object* (Bion, 1962b).

A practical aspect of this spectral view is that for social-ism to manifest, the psyche must renounce the possibilities inherent in *omnipotence* and *omniscience* (the narcissistic pole). There exists a significant symmetry (Chuster, 2018) between omnipotence and helplessness. All symmetries necessitate a myth or poetic language for broader expression, adopting the form of a *Language of Achievement* (Bion, 1970). I prefer to refer to it as the Language of Psychoanalytical Range (Chuster, 2023).

For instance, to socialize, an individual must abandon the belief in a singular explanation for facts. This belief replicates the infant's experience of being the center of the world, with the breast being always at their disposal. Without relinquishing this belief, which involves tolerating the frustration of incompleteness (principle of Uncertainty), human infants cannot successfully transition to another level of psychic experience, namely thinking. Thinking implies recognizing a link between oneself and two other people, acknowledging a tridimensional mind—the world of evolving vertices. Without embracing this concept, the prevalence of social-ism may never occur, and individuals will not benefit from the presence of a third person, starting with the father, extending to the family, and ultimately to society. Each entity plays a role that complements the mother's functions where she may be less adept.

Ethical-aesthetical principles express human capacities and limitations, serving as a constant reminder to critically evaluate our actions. They safeguard intuitive and imaginative work.

Bion's theory of *Oedipal pre-conception* offers a nuanced modification to Freud's discourse of the dissolution of the Oedipus complex. The ideas presented in Bion's *Transformations* (1965) emphasize the simultaneous creation and destruction of forms within the framework of three distinct container/contained configurations: commensal, symbiotic, and parasitic. This perspective implies that we encounter either evolution or involution but never dissolution, given the inherently Oedipal nature of the human mind. This evolutionary view about the Oedipus complex envisions the future of humanity in its growing capacity to cope with increasing disparities between individuals and their unique emotional experiences (Chuster 2018). I termed this as the *ethical-aesthetical principle of singularity*, emphasizing the undecidability of origins and the impossibility of resolving differences through elimination (Chuster 1999, 2002).

For example, certain patients believe that group formation necessitates the exclusion, devaluation, and eventual annihilation of the dissimilar. This *transformation in hallucinosis* disregards the singularity of an individual's internal group. Some patients engage in such behavior to involve the analyst in a conniving relationship, bypassing discussion and observation of the social representation of the individual. This highlights the complexity, necessitating the recognition of diverse perspectives and the eschewal of oversimplified resolutions.

Moreover, the establishment of an *ethical-aesthetical barrier*, based on trust and sincerity of words is paramount. This barrier cultivates a psychoanalytic character imbued with courage, compassion, and respect for life and truth (Chuster 2018). Certainly, respect for truth reinforces sincerity and trust. This might represent a circular argument, suggesting a proposition where each part depends on the veracity of the other. Circular arguments are often utilized to contemplate paradoxes, which lie at the heart of complex thinking.

The analyst is tasked with maintaining a mental state receptive to the turbulence of associated with the applications of *psychoanalytic objects* (Bion, 1962b). This requires reliance on their fluctuating *psychoanalytic function of personality*, which varies with the interaction of the Oedipal configuration and its evolution, indicating significant variability in analysts' capabilities, both across different analysts within the same analyst under varying circumstances.

Improving this ability, beyond personal analysis, involves maintaining a mental state as free as possible from *memory*, *desire*, and *the need for comprehension*. This implies observing the present moment devoid of pre-conceived notions from past ideas or desires for future outcomes. Bion's terms, while enigmatic, encourage us to continually reflect on our techniques for improvement.

The associative exercise with the Oedipus myth (Chuster, 1999, 2002, 2003, 2014, 2018) aids in developing intuition and the capacity to select an appropriate version (*language of achievement*, Bion, 1970) for use in the unfolding analytic process. Concurrent adherence to *ethical-aesthetical principles of observation* serves as a guiding principle (Chuster, 2002, 2003, 2014, 2018).

Notes

1 "A name used by *James Joyce*. In analysis certain ideas, whether expressed by analyst or analysand, are soon to provoke breeder-reactions; be it question or answer, it 'breeds' a whole range of new problems and ideas...." W.R. Bion, *A Memoir of the Future*, 1991, Karnac Books.

2 *Kurt Gödel Complete Works*, Volume I, 1986, Oxford University Press.

3 The Theory of Complexity often involves categorizing problems according to their level of difficulty to solve. Every problem has a specific class if the number of steps required for its solution is constrained by the problem's size. Additionally, assigning a problem to a complexity class allows for a non-deterministic solution.

4 E. Morin, *On Complexity*, 2008, Hampton Press, Cresskill.

5 E. Nagel & J. Newman, *Gödel's Proof*, 1958, Routledge Classics (2005 edition).

6 "Unless the analyst allows himself the exercise of his speculative imagination he will not be able to produce the conditions in which the germ of a scientific idea can flourish." W.R. Bion, *Taming Wild Thoughts*, 1997, Karnac Books.

Chapter 1

A Manifesto in Favor of Psychoanalytic Imagination

This chapter begins with a statement that has frequently recurred in my reflections, inspired by Bion's insights: Imagination unfolds through the engagement with challenging questions and the confrontation of the turbulent outcomes that arise in novel and unknown situations.

> When illumination occurs much depends on the years which discipline has been built up in the course of training and, more spontaneously, in dealing with frustration. Otherwise, the illumination is liable to initiate an uncontrolled reaction. For this reason progress in psychoanalysis can appear to precipitate a breakdown of frightening proportions. The illumination has often been described, usually in religious literature and by poets...[1]

To further elucidate and expand upon this notion, Plato's allegory of the cave[2] serves as a pertinent reference. In this philosophical tale, prisoners, chained to the walls, have spent their entire lives gazing at shadows cast by a bonfire behind them. Their perceptual world is confined to these fleeting silhouettes, as the shackles limit their ability to perceive the real world—a broader and unknown reality. Nevertheless, they are able to explain everything confined within the confines of their shadow-bound reality.

Plato's metaphor holds relevance across various contexts, including psychoanalytic practice. For psychoanalysts, the metaphorical chains consist of memory, desire, and the need for comprehension. These elements limit one of our most critical functions—the capacity to formulate questions, especially those unsettling ones that extend beyond what is readily observable. Therein lies the risk of becoming captives to our theories and constrained viewpoints, potentially reducing our ability to pose questions of genuine significance.

In *Attention and Interpretation*, Bion (1970) describes this hindrance as "*opacity*," a state where the emotions essential for a creative mind are replaced by activities to disperse anything related the pursuit of truth. This condition represents a form of intoxication with a deceptive essence, or a state of existence that trends towards not being present.

Let us now turn to the domain of science, which often grapples with such challenging questions, to explore the field of astrophysics.

DOI: 10.4324/9781003474128-2

The concept of time dilation becomes intriguing at high velocities. For instance, an astronaut traveling at 99.995% the speed of light to a star 650 light-years away would age only ten years upon return, while a thousand years pass on Earth, leaving everything familiar to him vanished.

While time travel to the past remains largely within a cinematic fiction, mathematicians propose its feasibility through "*closed timelike curves.*" Phenomena such as black holes, where time drastically slows—nearly halting—allow for the observation of the universe's inception, serve as good examples of those curves. This theory is profoundly comprehensive; what remains is developing the technology to make it a reality.

According to the Big Bang Theory,[3] our universe originated from a violent explosion at temperatures around 1027 degrees Celsius, expanding from a dense point of plasma radiation into everything observable today within three seconds.

Inspired by this, mathematicians[4] explored what preceded the Big Bang Theory. Through extensive calculations, they ultimately proposed that our universe began at the collapse of a star in a four-dimensional universe into a black hole—a singularity, from which our three-dimensional universe emerged.

We now encounter another intricate question: What exactly constitutes a four-dimensional universe? This concept remains elusive due to the inherent limitations of our imagination, rooted in our existence within a three-dimensional world. Yet, the ultimate challenge persists: How do we break through the confines of our imagination?

It is worth noting that imposing limits or establishing a caesura can be sufficient to spark the imaginative process, enabling us to break through its confines and tap into our intuitions. Bion highlights that this ability emerges when we can endure empty spaces, thereby expanding the field for infinite possibilities. This echoes what Keats referred to as *negative capability.*[5]

Similar to the scientists who dared to pose challenging inquiries, I propose that in psychoanalysis, we conclude our analytic sessions by asking: Have we presented our patients with uncomfortable questions today? Have we exposed further questions beyond those introduced by our patients?

The failure to ask these questions is obviously not indicative of a brain deficit or lack of intelligence. For instance, a rat's brain, though only as heavy as an olive, outperforms a cow's two-kilogram brain in intelligence. This raises the question: What distinguishes human intelligence? The key lies in our possession of smaller, more densely packed brain cells. Yet, this was not always the case for our distant ancestors. Over millions of years, a series of developments led to an increase in our brain's density. Tracing back approximately 8 million years, *Homo Habilis* had 40 billion brain cells, *Homo Erectus* 60 billion, and *Homo Sapiens* 86 billion neurons.

The leap from 60 to 86 billion neurons likely stemmed from the discovery of fire and its associated technologies, which allowed for faster calorie consumption to fuel the brain, which uses 20% of the calories consumed. The surplus time was then available for other activities, leading to enhanced intelligence. In contrast, an elephant's brain is fully occupied with finding food and maintaining stability due to its large body mass.

Nevertheless, our advanced brains may eventually hit a physical limit, potentially requiring the use of 100% of our brain cells. This would demand an evolutionary leap; otherwise, we risk stagnation like any other mammal.

Could there already be a *memoir* to this necessary future advancement? Are computers and cell phones precursors to this evolution?

Imagining further, if we were to use 100% of our brain capacity, we might need to develop an organic hard drive, enhanced by nanotechnology, that could not only boost our work capacity but also use nano cells to repair bodily failures. In about 150 years, it's conceivable that all our cells could be replaced with nano cells, which, powered by solar light, would eliminate the need for food, drink, or time-consuming bodily functions. This transformation could enable extended space travel, sustained by light alone, making traditional sustenance obsolete. Such advancements might finally enable us to comprehend a four-dimensional universe and, once again, dare to ask the same question: what preceded it?

Let us not underestimate our potential. We stand on the brink of becoming an interplanetary species, a dream that could become reality, for example, if an astronaut ventures to Mars to establish a human colony. Yet, despite these promising capabilities, we often direct our focus towards destructive behaviors on our own planet, causing harm to ourselves and the environment.

In the practice of psychoanalysis, certain patients frequently envision creating a personal refuge akin to Mars. This raises the question: Where does this metaphorical planet reside within their psyche or aspirations?

One patient in particular struggled with fear and anxiety about her emotions. She often resorted to dramatization, adopting various disguises, and crafting suspenseful stories. For instance, in one session, she arrived expressing concern over an upcoming job interview, pondering, "Will I present myself well? What if I stammer, or feel so overwhelmed that I lose my voice?" Such questions invariably evoked a heightened state of mental distress. When this anguish became unbearable, it threatened to fracture her mental functioning. In moments of despair, she lamented, "There is no place for me in the future."

I here quote Bion:

> Such fears can be seen in analysis of psychotic and claustrophobic patients. The Mad Hatter's tea party in *Alice in Wonderland* is a representation to which this timeless and spaceless "space" approximates.[6]

I will use Bion's representation of this fractured function (non-existent object) in *Transformations*:[7]

> It is feasible to interpret the patient's conflicting inclinations concerning her future. She attacks a 'fact' head-on, yet retreats from it, all the while maintaining an attachment to the 'fact' as a safeguard against the uncertainties and perils of life.

These tendencies may indeed harbor truth, albeit in contradiction. Consequently, the analyst serves as a container for both the feared object and the protective object, which appear incapable of coexisting within the same space. Absent is a third element to mediate the situation—the excluded third. Only the analyst's imaginative capacity, harnessed by intuition, can discover this absent element, thereby facilitating the emotional experience to unfold.

> In every case the emotion is to be part of the progression, breast → emotion (or place where breast was) → place where emotion was.[8]

In the initial stages of her analysis, the patient presented in a vigilant yet disorganized state, plagued by constant frustration. Despite complaints of extreme fatigue, multiple medical evaluations yielded no organic cause, ruling out a heart condition. The analyst observed a symmetry in these initial sessions: *excitement* on the end and *despair* on the other, often leading to claustrophobia, as illustrated by the following signs (Figure 1.1):

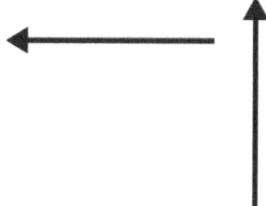

Figure 1.1 Broken Function.

The patient, having mastered the art of evasion, completely avoided experiencing anguish. Despite her visible tension, she consistently laughed to downplay the severity of her situation. This persistent laughter appeared to function as a survival technique. This prompted me to reflect on the nature of potential failures in her primary relationships. For instance, what might have been missing in her mother's reverie? Such hypothesis possibly pointing to certain impairments of the senses that offer the most primitive meanings.

Bion (1976) noted that the olfactory set functions as a receptor, measuring distances in a watery medium, suggesting it might be more stimulated in the embryonic mind than other senses. Consequently, it becomes plausible to hypothesize that this patient became adept at navigating social distances. Intimacy and sexual encounters induced "rhinitis," transforming a protective object into a persecutory one. One could speculate that her olfactory system is in constant search for predators in her surroundings. This surveillance function can extend to other senses, diminishing their sensitivity and effectiveness. As a result, her hearing might become dull, affecting her ability to assimilate or accurately understand interpretations.

A phobic situation, notably when linked to sexual contexts, points that the freedom to think is perceived as dangerous, as if exposing the individual to sexual perils. To mitigate this perceived threat, the patient attempts to restrict the analyst's freedom, inadvertently imposing similar constraints. This limitation becomes the primary source of her anguish, as the absence of freedom leads her thoughts towards death. As Spinoza[9] suggests, a free individual does not dwell on death.

This raises profound questions for us as analysts. Our focus typically spans small dimensions, such as the timeline of an individual, yet we also strive to delve into the distant past, exploring the earliest stages of mental life. However, what characterizes the mental life of a fetus, or how does a newborn's mental life evolve? What elements from these initial stages persist, influencing the present? Moreover, what mental disposition is required for us to embark on such exploratory journeys? In addition, at what pace should we proceed to reach these remote mental states?

I believe our exploration fundamentally depends on our imaginative capacity. The domain of thought in imagination is a space occupied by no-things; the space occupied by a particular no-thing marked by a sign.

> The attempt to free this domain from associations of space perception is supported by use of concepts such as 'thought' or 'thinking' or 'in the mind', but a thought continues to have the penumbra of associations proper to 'the place where...' the no-thing is.[10]

I will provide an example, reminiscent of a true story used as a model, in which the search for "no-things" leads one to undergo a distinct emotional experience of discovery that illuminates History.

In 1922, Howard Carter delved into the mysteries of the Valley of the Kings in Egypt. On the verge of abandoning his research, a worker drew his attention to a staircase of 16 steps carved into a rock, leading to an intact necropolis wall. On November 26, 1922, Carter breached the entrance to the tomb of Tutankhamun. Recounting that moment, he wrote:

> In the beginning, I could see nothing; the hot air that was coming from the room trembled the flame I was carrying. However, suddenly my eyes got used to darkness; details slowly came out, strange animals, statues made of gold. Everywhere gold was shining. For a moment, but for those who were behind me probably did feel like an eternity, my voice disappeared and when Lord Carnarvon asked me, *are you seeing anything?* The only words I found were, *yes. I can see stunning things.*[11]

The ancient Egyptians deeply revered their esteemed deceased, creating enduring artifacts during mourning. Inscriptions such as, "Oh night, open your wings over me like the eternal stars" adorned their sacred spaces.

Let us revisit our initial point of discussion. In Plato's allegory of the cave, a freed prisoner steps beyond the cave's confines into the external world, a transition marked by the pain of unaccustomed light. He faces a pivotal decision: to embrace the newfound light or return to the cave, potentially disturbing his former companions with accounts of the discomfort caused by the light.

Linking Plato's allegory[12] to Bion's notion of caesura invites several questions, including how we might free ourselves from the chains of memory and desire to see beyond our present dimension. Bion (1970) describes taking this step as the "Act of Faith," inspired by Nietzsche. Unlike religious faith, which accepts certain truths as absolute, the Act of Faith embodies a quest for creativity and an aspiration for the ineffable, unattainable truth. It involves embracing inherent uncertainties and the courage to ask unsettling questions, allowing for a playful exploration of words and their diverse meanings.

While religious faith typically entails adherence to established truths, reflecting an idealistic perspective (Platonism) and exhibiting a resistance to new ideas, favoring certainty, the *Act of Faith* is a wish for truth, representing a journey indispensable for mental development and insight.

This chapter concludes with a quotation from Bion:

On the way to being an analyst, you have to deserve the right to indulge your speculations, your speculative imagination. Perhaps you might want to sculpt, or paint, or draw, or compose music or fiction, in order to give your imagination an airing, to give it a chance to develop into something that might be scientific.[13]

Notes

1 W.R. Bion, *A Memoir of the Future*, 1991, Karnac Books.
2 Plato's allegory of the cave stands as one of the most renowned and insightful attempts to elucidate the essence of reality. The cave represents the common state of humanity, and the narrative of a dramatic exit from the cave serves as the origin of true understanding. Throughout the course of existence, every individual has, at some juncture, pondered variations of the same question: What is the purpose of our existence? What constitutes "reality," and what am I meant to do with (or about) it?
3 The Big Bang Theory serves as the prevailing cosmological model for the universe's inception and its subsequent large-scale evolution, outlining how the universe expanded from a state of extremely dense and high temperature. It offers explanations for a wide range of phenomena, such as the abundance of light elements, the cosmic microwave background, large-scale structure, and Hubble's Law. The singularity associated with the Big Bang, predicted by the known laws of physics at extreme densities, places the universe's age at about 13.8 billion years. Following its initial expansion, the universe cooled, allowing the formation of subatomic particles and simple atoms. These primordial elements formed massive clouds, coalescing through gravity within dark matter halos to create the stars and galaxies observed today.
4 Afshordi Niyaesh, Robert B. Mann, & Razieh Pourhasan, "Out of the White Hole: Origin for the Big Bang," *Journal of Cosmology and Astroparticle Physics*, Vol. 2014, April 2014.

5 "The capacity of the mind depends on the capacity of the unconscious—Negative capability. Inability to tolerate empty space limits the amount of space available." *The Complete Works of W.R. Bion*, Vol. 11, Chris Mawson (ed.), 2014, Karnac Books, p. 292.

6 W.R. Bion, *Transformations*, 1965, Karnac Books, p. 104.

7 W.R. Bion, *Transformations*, 1965, Karnac Books, p. 105, "Geometrical constructions have shown their value in representing the realizations found in geographical space." Proceeding with such an image of a broken function, I understand Bion to suggest that mathematical space may represent biological realities such as emotions.

8 W.R. Bion, *Transformations*, 1965, Karnac Books, p. 105.

9 Baruch Spinoza, *The Collected Work of Baruch Spinoza*, Edwin Curley (ed.), 2016, Princeton University Press.

10 W.R. Bion, *Transformations*, 1965, Karnac Books, p. 106.

11 Howard Carter, *The Discovery of Tutankhamun Tomb*, Vol. I, 2014, Bloomsbury.

12 John M. Coper (ed.), *Plato: Complete Works*, 1997, Hackett Publishing Company.

13 W.R. Bion, *Taming Wild Thoughts*, 1997, Karnac Books, p. 47.

Chapter 2

General Ideas on Transformations

From a psychoanalytic vertex, transformations are *emotional experiences*—a triangular configuration of links, represented as extreme abstractions denoted by the K, L, and H links.

> A theory of transformations must be composed of elements and constitute a system capable of the greatest number of uses (represented by the horizontal axis of the grid) if it is to extend the analyst's capacity for working on a problem with or without the material components of the problem present.[1]

Bion's theory of transformations expands upon Freud's Oedipal theory, providing valuable insights into a spectrum of mental states ranging from primitive to sophisticated. This theory reveals an unprecedented understanding of the depths of the mind and their socio-historical impacts. However, fully comprehending Bion's theory requires a paradigm shift in perspective towards his ideas.

Endorsed by Bion himself, the concept of transformations undeniably originated from the mathematical application of functions, an application coherent with his *A Theory of Thinking* (Bion, 1962a). Consequently, every transformation is a function within an infinite set that combines two elements to generate a third.

However, it is also important to explore the biological origins of mathematics, rather than attempting to impose a mathematical structure on biology, which stems from the mathematician's ability in identifying realizations that approximate to his constructs within the properties of the inanimate. Fundamentally, Bion represents biological realities, primarily emotions. His research on emotional experience (Bion, 1962b) sparked numerous conceptualizations, leading him to address transformations in the creative process of mental life.

As any creative process inevitably introduces turbulence, transformations involve examining the complexities of both the quantity and quality of turbulence in psychoanalytic work. By establishing a rule[2] for this observation, both in quality and quantity, it becomes possible to classify various types of transformations based on the intensity of turbulence.

In my point of view, the fundamental rules of observation in transformations might be found in a practical application of the *Catastrophe Theory*, initially

DOI: 10.4324/9781003474128-3

developed by the French mathematician René Thom[3] in 1959. The subsequent chapters explore this theory, as it is a key to understanding Bion's perspectives on transformations.

In many branches of mathematics, a transformation essentially implies a mathematical function that links sets, irrespective of its domain and codomain. Therefore, adhering to the basic principles of functions means linking elements inside a specific set or to another set. The term "transformation" might signify an exploration of, for example, the geometric aspects of a function with respect to invariants. This exploration necessitates functional analysis, which, in turn, requires a non-linear space, thus circling back to the study of transformations.

There is a clear difference between linear transformation and non-linear transformations. The former maintains a linear relationship between variables, preserving correlations unaltered within the transformation, while latter alters the relationship between variables, resulting in a different form with distinct movements in space.

The use of functions proved instrumental in conceptualizing every step in his book on transformations (Bion, 1965), serving as the concluding segment of a metaphorical bridge that both links and separates two crucial phases of his psychoanalytic exploration (Chuster, 2014, 2018).

Envisioning a bridge traversing the river of *complexity*, it navigates from a Kleinian-influenced path to Bion's self-explored road, where he develops several paradigmatic and epistemological points. The bridge's inception is anchored by the foundational pillar A—Bion's seminal paper, *A Theory of Thinking* (Bion, 1962a), referred to as the theoretical pillar. This pillar directs the bridge's trajectory through his subsequent works, *Learning from Experience* (Bion, 1962b) and *Elements of Psychoanalysis* (Bion, 1963), leading to the profound and unprecedented psychoanalytic deliberations in *Transformations* (Bion, 1965). This pivotal point marks the exit from the bridge, supported by the second pillar B, represented by the paper "Notes on Memory and Desire" (Bion, 1967), imaginatively termed as the technical pillar (Chuster, 2018) (Figure 2.1).

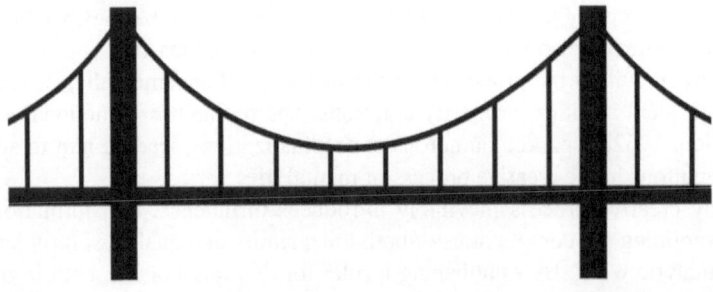

A. Theoretical pillar   B. Technical pillar

Figure 2.1

I use the metaphor of a bridge as a contemporary *pons asinorum* for Bion's readers. The term *"pons asinorum"* (bridge of asses)[4] was coined by Euclid in ancient Greece and served as a *sine qua non* condition for his students to advance their studies with him. Euclid originally challenged them to prove his fifth proposition concerning the repetition of angles in an isosceles triangle. Interestingly, this proposition had a colloquial sexual connotation at the time, alluding to an optimal angle for sexual intercourse. This double meaning led to jests from his students, compelling Euclid to change his challenge to proving the properties of the Pythagorean Theorem (Chuster, 2018).

Therefore, for those exploring Bion's theories on transformations and seeking to navigate this conceptual bridge without succumbing to confusion or disengagement, a solid grasp of certain mathematical and epistemological concepts, particularly the overarching concept of functions, is essential. It is beneficial to start with a basic comprehension of this central concept.

The mathematical concept of functions emerged in the 17th century alongside the development of calculus by Leibniz, who described how angles shift along a curve until reaching a certain point.

During the 17th century, the notion of functions was primarily understood as those defined by analytical expressions. The modern understanding of a function as a unique correspondence between sets was solidified through advancements in analytical mathematics by scholars like Weierstrass, Russell, and the introduction of the Theory of Infinite Sets by Cantor. These contributions were instrumental in redefining geometry through in terms of analysis.

The concept of a function is a cornerstone within mathematics, defining the relationship between two sets in which every element of the first set is associated uniquely with an element of the second set. This fundamental idea underpins a vast array of mathematical relationships and models, establishing it as a pivotal concept in both the study and application of mathematics.

Consider, for instance, the following illustrations:

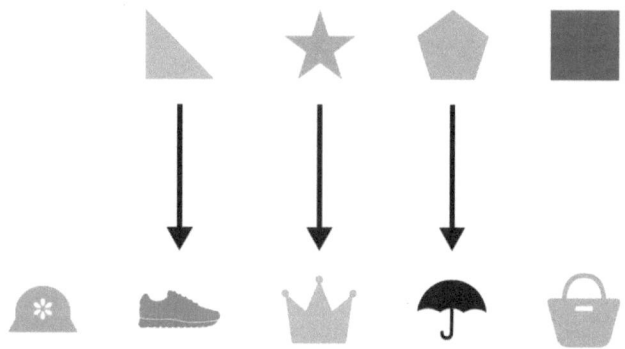

Figure 2.2

Figure 2.2 does not qualify as a function because there is no association between one of the elements (the square) of the upper set with any element in the lower set.

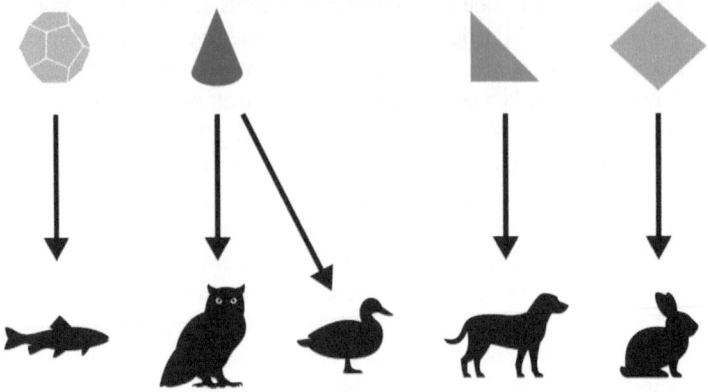

Figure 2.3

Figure 2.3 does not qualify as a function because one element (the cone) in the upper set is associated with more than one element in the lower set.

Now, consider the following example closely:

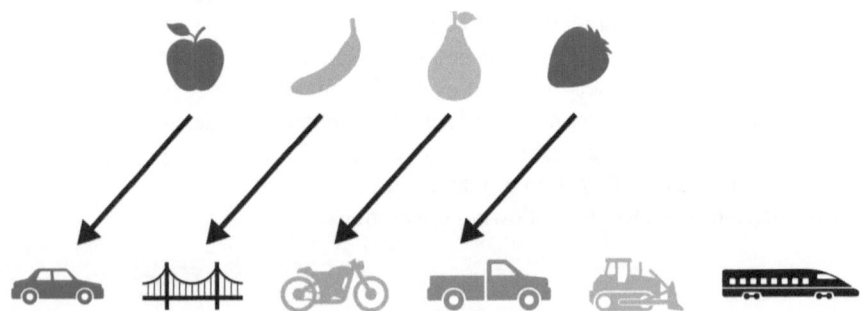

Figure 2.4

The interface in Figure 2.4 qualifies as a function because each element in the upper set is uniquely associated with only one element in the lower set. The presence of unmatched elements in the lower set does not compromise its status as a function.

This concept aligns with Bion's assertion, "An interpretation is a transformation; to display invariants, an experience, felt and described in one way, is described in another."[5]

In essence, for any two sets, A and B, the relationship between them is considered a function of A in B, if and only if, for every x in A, there exists a single y in B to which x is related (Figure 2.5).

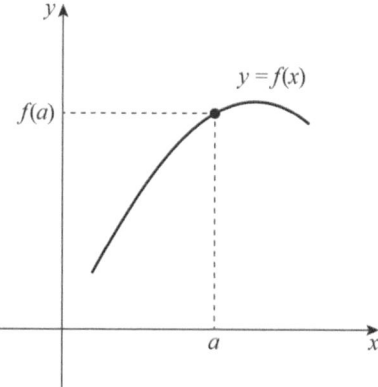

Figure 2.5 Graphics of a function.

The concept of function generalizes the traditional notion of mathematical formula, encapsulating singular mathematical links between two elements. A function can take various forms, such as equations, graphical representations, diagrams representing sets, rules of association, matching tables, and more. A function serves as a means to uniquely pair a function value (also known as a dependent variable) with each argument value (sometimes referred to as an independent variable).

Representing function-related pairs as points in a suitable space, like the Cartesian plane, emphasizes the requirement that each input (argument value) corresponds to a singular output (function value), visualized as a distinct point.

The concept of functions extends beyond calculus and numerical analysis. We intuitively employ this concept in various aspects of our daily lives whenever we link two elements. For instance, browsing a supermarket to find a specific item requires a function to correlate items with locations or items with prices.

Fundamentally, a function establishes a connection between a *domain* (a set of input values) with a *counter domain* or *codomain* (a set of output values), ensuring a precise association between each domain element and a codomain element. The set of codomain elements, for which there is at least one element in the domain to which it relates, is known as the set of images or the function image.

The concepts of *variables* (x) and *invariants* (f) are integral to the notion of a function, symbolically represented as f(x).

If we apply the concept of a function to psychoanalysis, Bion's fundamental theory of pre-conception illustrates a function where the invariant (f) is represented by ψ (Greek letter psi), and the variable element (x) is denoted by ξ (Greek letter ksi).[6]

$$\Psi\left(\xi\right) = f\left(x\right)$$

The analyst's role is manifested in providing interpretations, necessitating a capacity to articulate an integration of their senses, intuitions, conceptual understandings, and emotions in response to the patient's discourse. A pivotal concept introduced before transformations is the *psychoanalytic object*[7] (Bion, 1962b), which exemplifies a clear feature of complexity in Bion's thought, serving as a critical entry point in unraveling the implicit ideas in *Transformations* (Bion, 1965).

However, understanding Bion's text is always challenging, even for psychoanalysts who are open to accepting new ideas and paradigm shifts. The complexities within the text align with the "evolution" of an individual's personal journey, a nuance Bion explicitly emphasizes. Thus, the inherent difficulty in engaging with the book reflects its deliberate design. In navigating these challenges, the insights of the great Brazilian poet Mario Quintana[8] offer a form of enlightenment: "Stones on the way? I will take them all. One day I am going to build a castle."[9]

Notes

1 W.R. Bion, *Transformations*, 1965, Karnac Books, p. 39.
2 W.R. Bion, *Transformations*, 1965, Karnac Books, p. 93.
3 R. Thom, *Structural Stability and Morphogenesis*, 1972, NY University Press.
4 A bridge over a creek made of thin trunks of wood that animals cannot cross.
5 W.R. Bion, *Transformations*, 1965, Karnac Books, p. 4.
6 W.R. Bion, *Learning from Experience*, 1962b, Karnac Books, p. 69.
7 W.R. Bion, *Learning from Experience*, 1962b, Karnac Books, p. 68.
8 N. Facchinelli, *Mario Quintana, Vida e Obra*, 1976, Bels Editions.
9 Editor's note: This phrase is attributed to several poets, complicating the task of accurately determining its origin. Fernando Pessoa is also cited as a potential originator of the phrase. We chose to retain it as it eloquently captures the mindset of a reader who persists in engaging with *Transformations* despite the challenges posed by the text.

Chapter 3

Bion's Advanced Ideas on the Psychoanalytic Use of Functions

There is neither real evidence nor precise application for pure mathematical use of functions in psychoanalysis; therefore, the following ideas are likely to be *metaphors regarding* observations of human relationships. Thus, functions in psychoanalysis are akin to *mathematical poetry* describing the limits and possibilities of the psychoanalytic instrument known in Bion's work as the alpha function. In such poietic and linguistic context, the language of Transformations develops.

> The patient's relationship with himself is prejudiced if he cannot advance to recognition of a new experience and so falls back on existing meaning, or does progress and has to face frustration he cannot tolerate.[1]

Therefore, employing a function[2] model in psychoanalysis involves observing the relationship between the analyst and the analysand, and formulating hypotheses about their dynamics, identifying the invariants/variables within a particular context, and expanding the exploration to integrate elements through symmetry. This process incorporates a dual movement of integration and growth.

To work effectively with these parameters—namely invariants, variables, field, symmetry, and dual movement—identifying a construct capable of incorporating and integrating multiple variables is crucial. This approach broadens the scope for further integration. In analysis, this process is achieved by an enhanced employment of *Row C elements* (*dreams, myths, oneiric thoughts*), which strengthen the foundation for effective work with symmetric elements.

Figure 3.1 envisions the psychoanalyst's search for invariants within the positive area (+) with the intention to assimilate them into a cohesive construction. This process, inherently transformative, invariably includes a simultaneous destruction of forms within the negative area (−).

As observers, we can arbitrarily designate a starting point for transformation, subjectively marked as point **a** in Figure 3.1 (Tα). This trajectory advances towards point **b** (Tβ), representing the conclusion of transformation. Ultimately, the outcome involves both the creation and destruction of forms.

This phenomenon manifests as the concurrent existence of two distinct grids: a positive and a negative. It is important to recognize that the result of the process

DOI: 10.4324/9781003474128-4

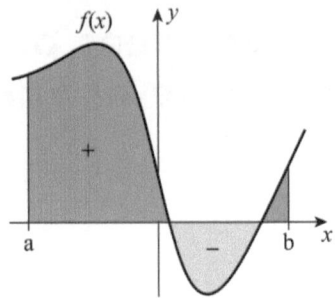

Figure 3.1 Trajectory of Transformation.

(represented by x) is relatively limited in comparison with the entire spectrum of movement. This implies that despite the considerable effort invested in a session, the final impact remains comparatively modest.

The outcome may further diminish, become null, or even transition to a negative state if negative elements predominate. In other words, patients predominantly influenced by the psychotic part of their personality are more inclined to generate a Negative Grid.[3] In contrast, a patient with a predominantly non-psychotic personality is more likely to engage in constructive activities that promote the development of the K link.

In practice, this implies that analysts, irrespective of whether the patient articulates complaints, can become targets of grievances, with frustration serving as an invariant. These complaints, despite their various manifestations (variables), are consistently present. They may be implicit or explicit, mild or intense, and their nature is discernible through the type of transformation (Bion, 1965).

Subtle complaints may facilitate discussion and insight, whereas those originating from the negative end of the spectrum can manifest as resentful, critical, cruel, hostile, or derogatory criticisms. These more severe manifestations are transformations in hallucinosis.

Figure 3.2 outlines functions where Y represents the analysand and may represent a component of a function within a specific field. F(x) represents the analyst's alpha function, which must be attuned to the analysand, as indicated by F(x) = Y. This formula illustrates that both the analysand and the analyst contribute to the formation of the analytic function.[4]

When working with transformations in the psychoanalytic process, employing *C elements* (*dreams, myths, oneiric thoughts*) to create analogies for transference observations offer many advantages; these elements become essential. In Figure 3.2, the point "**a**" marks the beginning of the analyst's creative state of mind, characterized by no memory and desire, akin to a state of negative capability. In this state of observation, the analyst begins to capture variables and invariants until reaching a constant conjunction. At this moment, the analyst may decide, for instance, to offer an interpretation of the patient's invariants (Y). It is important to note that

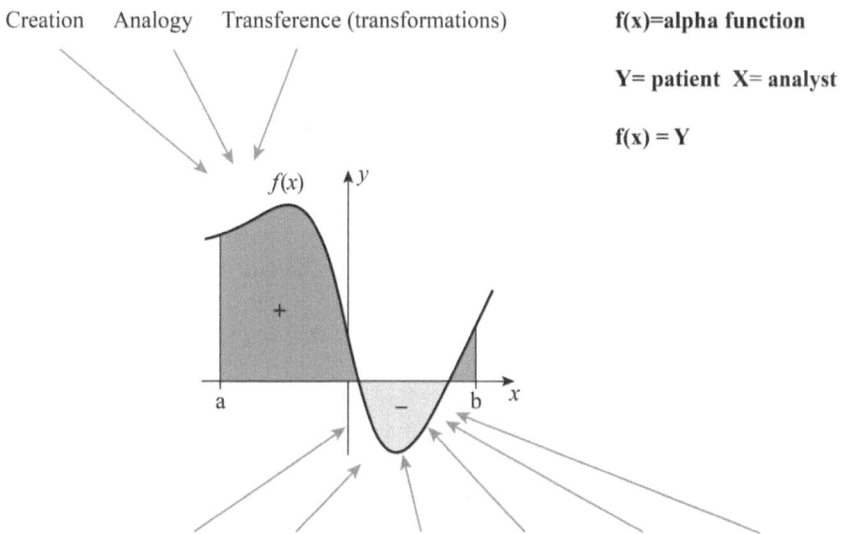

Figure 3.2

a constant conjunction is a function of the observer's consciousness; therefore, it varies according to the number of elements perceived by the observer. This characteristic is typical of a realm where uncertainty is unavoidable.

In Bion's advanced Grid (Bion, 1970), the evolution of *Ta* (analyst) should be a consequence, and it is noteworthy that the creative activity decreases as the analogy transitions into an interpretation.

The *C elements* serve as psychoanalytic anchors for the analyst's interpretations that would ideally contain the emergence of elements of a Negative Grid. However, the critical determining factor between the paths of growth and decay always lies within the link. These paths are inherently at odds due to the radical opposition of their objectives. Take for example, the relationship between the mouth and the breast; growth is contingent upon the significance of their link, which must outweigh the importance of each individually. Conversely, should the importance assigned to either the mouth or the breast exceed the other, we encounter degeneration/non-integration instead of growth/integration.

Every birth, physical or psychological, emerges from a disagreement between the container and the contained, representing a *caesura*. Therefore, as psychoanalysis continually deals with such caesuras, recognizing and leveraging these disagreements become crucial. This process relies on the capacity (alpha function) to create a bridge between two elements or functions, thereby establishing an analytical field where the integration of invariants and variables is operational. This requires the application of the concept of symmetry.[5] However, at this point, one of the paramount challenges in analysis arises: the communication between a dynamic personality with another dynamic personality, implying that variables are in constant flux. This reality anchors us in a domain marked by constant uncertainties and incompleteness.

Figure 3.2 illustrates the consistent emergence of negative elements, signifying the destruction of forms, throughout the integration processes. At the end of the negative trajectory within the analytic space, we have *asymmetry* and degeneration, invariably due to the dominance of one of the objects over the link.

Bion illustrates this dynamic through the case of a patient with stammering, whose development was "detained" by the disproportionate importance placed on physiological functions (urinating and defecating). For this patient, the mouth became an object requiring continual gratification by the tongue, preventing the formation of meaningful relationships.

Through stammering, the patient represented an omniscient relationship with his body, imposing a significant barrier in communication. He projected his experience of this limitation onto his relationships, particularly with his children. The stammerer restricts his audience when struggling to articulate words, generating a circularity when the interlocutor fails to understand his speech. This dynamic further illustrates an intrapsychic link where one function, specifically speech, overpowers another, thereby affecting the relationships among all aspects of the Self. This includes mental functions, such as thinking, and the connection with the body.

In psychoanalytic practice, we encounter various forms of stammering. For instance, stammering may manifest as a restrictive relationship with the analyst, wherein the patient perceives themselves as inferior, due to a top-bottom, moralistic logic. In this dynamic, the patient might view the analyst as an authority figure who imposes limitations, casting them into the role of a humiliated and subordinate child. Such a dynamic can lay a powerful foundation for *transformation in hallucinosis*, where "stuttering" distorts the perception of time, rendering it fragmented and erratic. The outcome underscores a moralistic logic driven by the cruelty of the superego and rivalry with "O."

The interpretations or constructions formulated by the analyst should embody an intuitive link between the analyst and the analysand. This link develops through the analyst's creative imagination and the analysand's capacity to dream and comprehend (alpha function of both parties). Yet, the link remains perpetually vulnerable to deliberate attacks and is inherently weakened and strained by the limited outcomes achieved. Once again, it is crucial to underscore the necessity for the protection and maintenance of the link.

Figure 3.3 illustrates the development of an interpretation in an *Advanced Grid* (Bion, 1970). The shaded area represents *C elements* integrated by the alpha function, $f(x)$, within the transformation field. Although the illustration employs mathematical terms, it signifies not precision but approximations of a selected fact. The process begins with the selection of one aspect of the patient for analytic observation, thus marking the inception of the transformation. This step begins with the collection of field variables, which are subsequently united by the selected fact,[6] culminating at point (b), where the transformation ends.

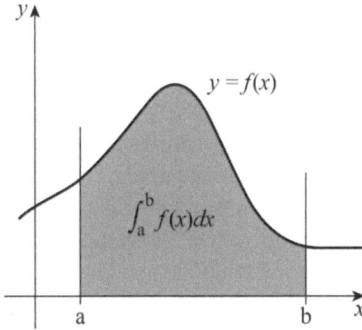

Figure 3.3 Development of Interpretation.

Figure 3.4 illustrates the field created by transformations between the analyst and the analysand.

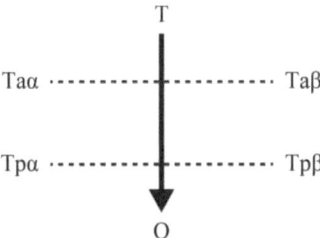

Figure 3.4 Psychoanalytic Field.

T	Transformation
Taα	The point where the analyst's transformation begins
Taβ	The point where the analyst's transformation ends
Tpα	The point where the patient's transformation begins
Tpβ	The point where the patient's transformation ends
O	The emotional experience of the session (the thing-in-itself)

Before proceeding, it is pivotal to revisit one key question: how to protect the development of interpretation?

The answer to this question involves employing reflections and corresponding intuitions to create a Grid after a session, which would serve as a crucial instrument for mental training, akin to mental gymnastics (Bion, 1977a). This ensures that analysts remain adept and prepared to tackle the inherent challenges of analytic work. Designed for personal reflection after sessions, the Grid enables analysts to process session material without the direct pressure or criticism from the analysand. This practice is vital for enhancing the analyst's capacity to form analogies and navigate the complexities of the analytic process.

The value of practicing with the Grid becomes more pronounced for psychoanalysts when working with patients whose communication is restricted to a limited range. In such cases, the analyst faces a dichotomy: the patient resonates either with the precisely correct communication or with nothing at all. Thus, precision in interpreting communications becomes critical, necessitating the analyst to adopt a more expansive toolset. Employing symmetry can facilitate access to this wider spectrum. However, this raises the question: Which elements ensure this quality if selection is possible?

One solution is to capture and utilize the *language of emotions* in analytical constructions, given that emotions inherently possess mathematical accuracy.[7] Yet, a prevalent challenge with such patients is their inability to endure psychic pain, leading them to strip emotions from their communications through broad generalizations or narrow particularizations—signifying the presence of *beta elements*.

For instance, a female patient interpreted a series of failures in her unsuccessful romantic engagements as proof of her own omnipotence, maintaining an omniscient conviction of her destructive impact on others through a generalization: "All my relationships fail." Yet, this perspective does not apply to her professional achievements, where she received ample respect from colleagues. One might raise the question: What causes this splitting? What leads her to focus on an obstinate negative self-view while disregarding her positive attributes?

Over several sessions, it became evident that the patient was trying to maintain a considerable emotional distance from the analyst, seemingly to shield him from her potentially destructive power. This distancing appears to be achieved through the employment of monotonous generalizations and a constant false courtesy.

Deprived of the emotional content, the analyst finds it challenging to accomplish the necessary precision in interpretations. This situation, as depicted using one of Bion's metaphors (1977), is like an elephant lumbering after a tiger. The metaphor captures a predator/prey dynamic where the prey (the tiger, the unconscious) remains elusive. In such a scenario, the analyst may find himself cast in the role of an ineffective predator, resembling an elephant: cumbersome, sluggish, ill-suited, with a profound self-view as the least competent analyst, as their interpretations fail to breach the patient's emotional gap. Bion (1979) suggests viewing this feeling as a gift from the patient, advising to make the best of a bad job.

Bion (1977) shares his own experience with this situation, most notably with a musician who sought the perfect note, and another patient whose acute visual sensitivity made any deviation from the perceived correct color unbearable.

An occasional spectator once told me about witnessing a violin lesson led by the renowned Isaac Stern,[8] exclusively for a select group of accomplished American violinists, focusing on Brahms's Violin Concerto. Stern played a passage, which the violinists then attempted to replicate. From the spectator's non-professional perspective, their imitation seemed accurate, but Stern insisted otherwise, highlighting errors with each repetition. As the violinists attempted to replicate Stern's performance, his frustration grew with each repetition. He criticized their efforts, suggesting they were fundamentally incorrect, as though they lacked the basic understanding of violin playing.

Frustration mounted until one violinist protested, "That's enough, stop with this nonsense. We are not you. We are not Isaac Stern!" The outburst startled Stern, as if awakening from a dream, offering a humble apology. An observer explained that the contention centered on the unique pressure Stern applied to a string for a specific note (Fa sharp), a subtlety tied to his unique physicality.

A fruitful discussion of this incident revolves around the burden imposed by singularity—despite overarching similarities, there exists a tipping point where the weight of minor differences can become overwhelmingly significant.

The concept of sincerity also emerges as vital in psychic development. Bion, navigating the intricacies of psychoanalytic technique, emphasizes the significance of moving beyond the evidence solely provided through verbal language, echoing Freud's warning about symbolic disguises. Yet, Bion ponders the appropriate response to symbolic revelations. Particularly in children, these symbolic expressions often constitute the primary mode of communication, aligning with their developmental cognitive capacities, typically offering a more direct and revealing form of expression than that of adults.

Adult patients may shield themselves by avoiding the candor required in the analytic process, perhaps due to a lack of trust in the psychoanalyst or their interpretations. They may conceal their genuine feelings behind their words, giving the impression of agreeing with the interpretations. Subtle manifestations of this problem can be detected through nuanced revelations, highlighting the intricate challenges in establishing a genuine and transparent therapeutic relationship.

As analysts—not linguists or philologists—we frequently reveal hidden meanings of words or present a new perspective through interpretations to our patients. This process often evokes a simultaneous sense of surprise and appreciation. In such moments, patients commonly respond with statements like, "Oh, I had never thought of that before." Freud considered this as a subtle form of affirmation, proposing that it was a translation of, "Yes, at least this time, you (the analyst) are correct about my unconscious."

However, it is crucial not to deceive ourselves, as a Negative Grid exists simultaneously, where the denial of the analyst's creativity, fueled by jealousy or envy, becomes apparent. For instance, a patient might non-verbally convey, "I never imagined this could be thought without my thinking it first," indicating a belief in the originality of their thought above all others. Is this illusion a feature of the social group to which the patient belongs? In other words, is it a social illusion?

Additional questions arise: To what extent does the patient employ projective identification, potentially transforming the illusion into a delusion? Could this evolve into a delusion of grandiosity or megalomania, transformation in hallucinosis? If so, what destructive impact might this transformation in hallucinosis have on the patient's relationships, similar to the case previously presented? Alternatively, is there evidence of a previous "breakdown" now manifesting in financial procedures, corruption, and social status?

Bion draws attention to yet another symbolic disguise, one that is intricately woven into the fabric of our everyday life—money. The adage that money is the world's spring is a logical belief, grounded in habits that can potentially transform the use of money into a sense of omnipotence. This transformation is rooted in the idea that engaging in financial rituals can effectively alleviate anxieties related to dimensions of time and space. In this context, some patients might believe their financial capacity alone qualifies them to "acquire" and "sustain" analysis. These beliefs require further exploration.

A practical approach might begin with a direct inquiry, asking how the patient envisions sustaining analysis without addressing the part of themselves that actively resists living a life that is worth living. How alive does the patient feel in his time and space? What is the cost of an analysis? Conversely, what might be the cost of not having an analysis?

These questions explicitly underscore the issues explored in this chapter, which are facets of Bion's basic theory of pre-conception and transformations. This theory, repeatedly illustrated throughout this book, presents pre-conception as the inherited foundation of human search for knowledge. It prompts us to seek out a mind—initially that of the mother—as a means for survival. In its most abstract form, pre-conception is a function that indicates humans' existence within the dimensions of time and space, with existence gaining significance because of these two dimensions.

Disconnections between these dimensions, often instigated by the dominance of the psychotic part of the personality, are akin to a broken function. This clinical situation finds an analogy with *"existing objects."* He describes this broken function as *"violent, greedy and envious, ruthless, murderous and predatory, without respect for the truth, persons or things."*[9] One may view it as a raw representation of the Mother Nature, whose sole function is to search for existence. This perception can be very daunting, especially as it overthrows all notions of omnipotence.

Bion says,

> It is, as it were, what Pirandello might have called a Character is Search of an Author. In so far as it has found a 'character', it appears to be a completely immoral conscience. This force is dominated by an envious determination to possess everything that objects that exists possess including existence itself.[10]

Pirandello's discourse on art illustrates how art and illusion intertwine with reality, emphasizing the subjective nature of perception where words are unreliable and reality is both true and false simultaneously. His tragic farces are often viewed as forerunners for the theatre of the absurd:

> The man, the writer, the instrument of the creation will die, but his creation does never die. And to live forever, it does not need to have extraordinary gifts or to be able to work wonders. Who was Sancho Panza? Who was Don Abbondio? Yet they live eternally because—live germs as they were—they had the fortune to find a fecundating matrix, a fantasy which could raise and nourish them: make them live forever.[11]

Nature can be feared as a contradictory object in the eyes of humans. It is a name given to an entity, sometimes outside, sometimes inside. It has been an object of observation since the beginning of time. Fear of Nature seems to govern the existence of characteristics described above in the mind of the patient, who appears to entertain the phantasy of such a contradictory object.

But the patient may identify himself with such an object and the contradiction then lies in his existing sufficiently to feel that he does not exist. The rule that a thing cannot both be and not be is inadequate.[12]

Notes

1 W.R. Bion, *Transformations*, 1965, Karnac Books, p. 54.
2 Nikolai K. Nikolski, *Operators, Functions, and Systems: An Easy Reading*, The American Mathematical Society, 2002.
3 Arnaldo Chuster, *A Lonesome Road, Essays in the Complexity of W.R. Bion's Work*, 2014, Trio Studio Graphics Digital, Brazil. The author explains "The initial premise of the Negative Grid is to evaluate psychic development based on the creation of Lies," p. 161.
4 Andranik S. Tangian and Joseph Gruber (eds.), *Constructing and Applying Objective Functions*, 2002, Springer.
5 Symmetry is used in accordance with Matte Blanco's definition of this concept. See Chapter 10 for more details.
6 Henri Poincare, *Science and Method*, translated by Francis Maitland, 2007, Cosimo Inc., p. 30.
7 Arnaldo Chuster, *Language of Psychoanalytical Range*, 2023, Hedges Publishers.
8 Isaac Stern, *My First 79 Years*, written with Chaim Potok, 2001, Da Capo Press.
9 W.R. Bion, *Transformations*, 1965, Karnac Books, p. 102.
10 W.R. Bion, *Transformations*, 1965, Karnac Books, p. 102.
11 Luigi Pirandello, *Six Characters in Search of an Author*, Dover Publications Inc. (edition 1998), p. 6.
12 W.R. Bion, *Transformations*, 1965, Karnac Books, p. 102.

Chapter 4

Catastrophic Change

The concept of catastrophic change, introduced in the first chapter of the book *Transformations* (Bion, 1965), is a comprehensive notion covering all transformations described by Bion. Therefore, it is essential to consider psychoanalysis within the spectrum of transformations.[1]

> In this situation the analyst must search the material for invariants to the pre and post-catastrophic stages. These will be found in the domain represented by the theories of projective identification, internal and external objects.[2]

The term "catastrophe" derives from the Greek "*katastrophe*," meaning a "sudden overturn" or a "shift in expectations." Specifically, "*kata*" translates to "down," and "*strophein*" to "turning upside down." Generally, it denotes a sudden shift in the pattern of an event.

The terms "trigger," "event," and "pattern" articulate the sequence of perceptions associated with a catastrophic change. Observations include elements both before and after certain events, termed pre- and post-catastrophic states. In subsequent writings, Bion (1975) refers to this as a "caesura," a critical juncture, an extremely fluid entity that bridges these states, which will be explored in depth in later chapters.

A catastrophe is an alteration of a specific state. Common examples include sudden stock market crashes, rain-induced landslides, tsunamis, an instant transition from darkness to light upon flipping a switch, or the reverse when darkness ensues. It is important to recognize that catastrophes can be either destructive or productive. I propose labeling the destructive instances as "calamities" and reserving the term "catastrophic changes" for the productive ones.

The states of water, from stillness to ice, boiling, or steam, exemplify productive catastrophic changes, corresponding to four transformations. By defining a specific field and taking into account the effects of changes beyond this field, we identify six types of transformations as outlined by Bion. Therefore, the initial transformation involves establishing a specific field, the final transformation relates to the impacts extending outside the field, and four types of transformations occur within the field.

DOI: 10.4324/9781003474128-5

In psychoanalysis, treated as the specific field, mental states can be depicted through a triangle, at the heart of which lies the Oedipal theory. During analysis, the psychoanalyst observes facts within an emotional experience (Bion, 1962b). This triangle (see Figure 4.1), symbolizing the experience, can undergo a vertex change within the same quadrant, representing a transformation in knowledge (K). If it moves to another quadrant while maintaining its properties, it constitutes a transformation in rigid motion. A hyperbolic process that enlarges or reduces the experience in a different quadrant indicates a projective transformation. Lastly, a logical inversion in an opposite quadrant, aligning with a moralistic theory, signifies a transformation in hallucinosis.

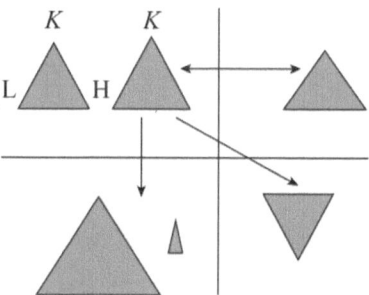

Figure 4.1 Four Types of Transformation.

The French mathematician René Thom developed qualitative mathematical models initially named "Models of Morphogenesis." Later, he introduced the term "Catastrophe Theory"[3] to describe these models more accurately.

In psychoanalysis, the application of Catastrophe Theory enables us to focus on non-linear observations, facilitating a form of alignment or symmetry among numerous potential outcomes. In projective geometry, this model can be loosely explained by Desargues' theorem (Bion, 1975), which discusses bundles of parallel lines converge at infinity. Meanwhile, triangular configurations reveal symmetries when related to a central axis, which briefly acts as a guiding principle (Figure 4.2).

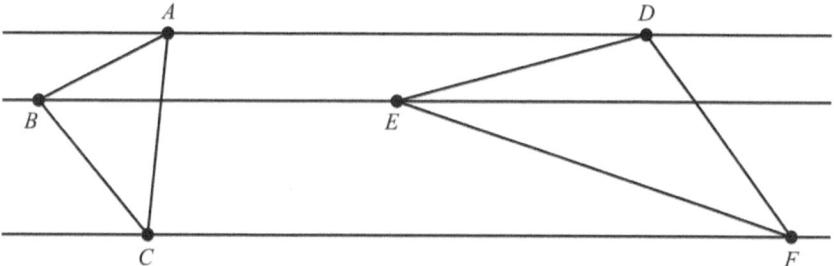

Figure 4.2

Using the theorem as an analogy for the relationship between analyst and analysand, the central axis links the analyst's Oedipal configuration with that of the analysand. This link signifies a potential for catastrophic change.

Bion (1977b) illustrates this concept of "psychoanalytic geometry" by proposing a spectrum. This spectrum was used in the previous chapter to illustrate the activity of a psychoanalytic function:

Creation → *analogy* → *transference* → *illusion* → *group delusion* →
delirium → *hallucination* → *asymmetry* → *degeneration*

The foremost challenge in comprehending the mathematical depiction of the world hinges on the nuanced interplay between continuous and discontinuous phenomena. Often, the line distinguishing continuity from discontinuity is so fine that observing them requires specific conditions, mainly due to their singularities. Psychoanalysts face a parallel scenario. Although theoretical frameworks like Freud's concept of transference exist to study these phenomena, discreet phenomena may go unnoticed if the psychoanalyst lacks preparedness. Integrating these underlying concepts into transformations could generate a novel perspective on psychoanalysis.

Although Bion did not have explicit access to the scientific and mathematical theories of catastrophic changes, his exceptional intuition enabled him to weave them into the fabric of psychoanalytic thought. This integration is evident in Bion's advocacy for using functions (1962b, 1963, 1965) as the primary means to observe and understand transformations within the psychoanalytic domain.

The application of functions suggests that living entities are marked by numerous singularities, a complex idea embodied in Bion's psychoanalytic object (1962b) through the factor (μ), representing the vicissitudes of a biological object. This concept spans a wide spectrum of possibilities, from minor adjustments to major life catastrophes like illness or death.

Drawing insights from Catastrophe Theory does not necessarily pave the way to investigative success or offer a blueprint for survival. More often, it highlights the recognition of our limitations. Yet, this realization is as an acknowledgment of the constant flux inherent in all things over time.

The *Psychoanalytic Object* (Bion, 1962b) exemplifies an object in perpetual flux. Its observation requires a continuous stream of creative thoughts to remain abreast. Fundamentally, it entails reconciling our imaginative conjectures with rational ones, recognizing a caesura created by this ever-evolving object.

To reiterate the core concept, Catastrophe Theory elucidates the interplay of continuous and discontinuous phenomena, leading to constant turbulence and singularities. Bion, akin to mathematicians, employed this conceptual framework to observe the unconscious, thereby introducing a novel perspective in thinking. This approach resulted in changing the terminology from conscious to finite and from unconscious to infinity.

In the past four decades, the theory of singularities has evolved to a sophisticated level, primarily due to the contributions of H. Whitney, J. Mather,[4] and R. Thom. This theory has emerged as a potent analytical tool across various scientific fields, especially in conjunction with the theory of bifurcation, an idea initially put forward by Poincaré and expanded upon by the Russian mathematician A. Andronov.

Edgar Morin, a contemporary thinker, delved deeply into the singularities articulated by Whitney and Thom, articulating their essence through his complexity theory. At times, these concepts blur the lines with poetry or philosophy, making it difficult to discern their veracity. The question of whether they serve merely as constructs to mitigate the fear of the unknown associated with ignorance is worth asking. Yet, Poincaré suggested that mathematicians do not eliminate obstacles; they relocate them to a frontier for discussion, often on an unconscious level. One hopes that psychoanalysts will embrace a similar methodology.

Bion (1965, 1970) advocated for a broad discourse to shed light on these matters. From the dawn of humanity, human observations have emerged in three primary fields: art, science, and religion, each striving to depict and grasp the essence of human nature and the natural world. Within these realms, certain individuals have consistently distinguished themselves by their capacity to notice what remains invisible to most. Frequently, they identified what was plainly in sight, yet embedded within such observations was something exceedingly rare: *a memoir of the future.* They act as illuminators, embodying the simplest form of catastrophic change by turning on the light.

In the realm of religion, such visionaries are known as mystics, while in art and science, they are celebrated as geniuses. This latter term underscores the interconnectedness of science and art, suggesting a symmetrical relationship between the two. Regardless of the terminology, these figures create emotional turbulence (Bion, 1976) within the societal fabric through the impact of their groundbreaking ideas.

The influence of a genius is sometimes immediately recognized as a pivotal epistemological shift in history; other times, these shifts may take years, or even generations, to be acknowledged or understood.

Leonardo da Vinci, in what Bion (1975) refers to as moments of decision/creation, depicted spiral hair in his drawings as a symbol of this turbulence, signaling transitions from one mental state to another, akin to illuminating darkness. Leonardo, despite his disciplined approach, often framed his sketches within a circle or field, setting boundaries for his creative explorations.

John Milton, in *Paradise Lost*, explores turbulence through the Invocation of Light, viewed from the perspective of Satan. He describes the emergence of the world from deep and dark waters, a theme of creation wrested from the void.

The aforementioned creators did not begin with clear objectives. Instead, they ventured into the unknown, letting their imagination navigate. Leonardo's sketches represent the early gestation of creative ideas—internal movements in search of an author, often requiring interpreters to unveil their singularities.

Paul Klee, initially setting out to create a political cartoon featuring German Kaiser, ended up with *Angelus Novus*, a piece that Walter Benjamin interpreted as symbolizing the Angel of History, depicting an angel propelled by the winds of History, witnessing the growing distance from Heaven and a trail of devastation.

Michelangelo, in his later years, revisited and brought to life ideas from his youth, exemplified by his creation of the statue of David.

Milton's work, veiled as a biblical text and intended as social and political critique, transcended its original aim, inspiring a wealth of poetic energy and interpretations across literary epics by authors such as Cervantes, Camus, and Shakespeare, thus transforming political commentary into transcendent poetry. Interestingly, *Paradise Lost* is a metaphor for the embryonic mind giving birth to the human essence.

Biblical and mythological narratives also illustrate the need for intermediaries in conveying profound truths. Moses had Aaron, Krishna guided Arjuna, and in mythology, figures like Automedon served as crucial links between divine will and human action.

Similarly, apostles propagated Jesus' teachings, each interpreting divine messages for humanity. This highlights the transformative power of visionary insight across various domains of human thought and creativity.

Isaac Luria, a Kabbalistic mystic, chose not to write down his teachings, citing a perceived lack of emotional depth in written words. Nevertheless, his disciples documented his ideas, which intriguingly resemble early concepts of quantum physics as applied to astronomy. This raises the question: Could Luria have had a premonition of the future of science. He claimed regular conversations with the prophet Elijah to explore profound doctrines, and during sleep, his soul would ascend to heaven to converse with great masters.

Vincent van Gogh, the renowned Dutch painter born in 1853, depicted turbulence in works like "Starry Night" (1889), where spirals of light and clouds seem to animate the canvas, mirroring natural turbulence seen in fluids and gases. This prompts speculation: Could he have anticipated the imagery of a star field captured by the Hubble Space Telescope in 2004, with its swirling dust and gas? While it is tempting to draw such parallels, in psychoanalytic practice, the aim is not to chase an elusive truth but to encourage dialogue and provide a space for thoughts and emotions.

Meister Eckhart, a pivotal figure in medieval philosophy, mysticism, and Neoplatonism, delivered sermons rich with paradoxes. His unique use of language often necessitated interpretation, sometimes leading to misinterpretations. At the end of his life, he faced an inquisition trial.

These instances highlight the myriad ways in which images, characters, and personal experiences can embody and convey emotional turbulence, subsequently interpreted by society and individuals. Yet, psychoanalysts typically focus more modestly on the clinical aspects of these dynamics.

Notes

1 W.R. Bion, *Transformations*, 1965, Karnac Books, p. 4.
2 W.R. Bion, *Transformations*, 1965, Karnac Books, p. 9.
3 René Thom, *Structural Stability and Morphogenesis*, 1975, W. A. Benjamin.
4 J. Damon, "John Mather's Pioneering Work in Singularity Theory and Its Enduring Legacy," Conference in Memory of John N. Mather, October 1–3, 2018, Taplin Auditorium, Princeton University.

Chapter 5

Why Only Four Transformations Inside the Psychoanalytic Field?

The question posed by this chapter's title is the application of René Thom's Catastrophe Theory, which was explored in the previous chapter. This theory postulates that within any dynamic system, there are only four types of transformations: one involving rigid motion and three involving non-rigid motion transformations. This categorization coincides with Bion's descriptions, despite no evidence that Bion directly referenced Thom's theory. This coincidence suggests that Bion might have arrived at his insights intuitively, potentially drawing from sources that paralleled Thom's work.

> It is not knowledge of reality that is at stake, nor yet the human equipment for knowing. The belief that reality is or could be known is mistaken because reality is not something which lends itself to being known. It is impossible to know reality for the same reason that makes it impossible to sing potatoes; they may be grown, or pulled, or eaten, but not sung. Reality has to be "been": there should be a transitive verb "to be" expressly for use with the term "reality.[1]

> The spoken word seems significant only because it is invisible and intangible; the visual image is similarly significant because it is inaudible. Every word represents what is not—a 'no-thing,' to be distinguished from 'nothing.'[2]

In this chapter, to avoid redundancy in discussing this theory and its applications, the focus will be on elaborating the four transformations within the psychoanalytic field. Additionally, I will extend the discussion with supplementary information and provide a personal perspective.

5.1   Transformations in Hallucinosis

These transformations take place at the juncture where the capacity for thought begins to disintegrate. Bion, without explicitly defining the term, seems to have introduced "hallucinosis" to differentiate it from hallucinations—sensory experiences associated with psychoses. Hallucinosis, therefore, denotes singularities in the domain of thought.

DOI: 10.4324/9781003474128-6

The degree of distortion in hallucinosis that influences thought processes convey a moralistic logic, predisposed by two main factors: the cruelty of the superego and rivalry with "O." Both elements are capable of undermining life values,[3] initiating a process designed to validate a false premise. The most detrimental outcome of this process could be the establishment of a belief system in which lies are considered more desirable and safer than seeking the truth. Other possible false premises might involve asserting that actions are more important than words or believing in one's superiority over others. Despite being founded on false premises, these moralistic logics might superficially appear to be correct. Therefore, to break the cycle of transformations in hallucinosis, interpretations must expose the fallacy of the underlying premise; failing to do so renders any dialogue with the deceptive logic a futile endeavor.

5.2   Projective Transformations

These transformations establish links between meanings that have not yet been explicitly expressed in verbal language. There is a subliminal prevalence of projective identification over verbal language. These transformations often present meanings through verbal actions that do not express feelings, thereby, making them more readily perceptible as hyperboles. A frequent example found in patients' speech is the elaborate recounting of daily life's concrete details, as opposed to conveying their struggles or emotions during the session. At times, these hyperboles can induce feelings of drowsiness or lethargy in the analyst.

> The analyst's transformations employ the vehicle of speech just as the musician's transformations are musical and the painter's pictorial. Though the analyst attempts to transform O, in accordance with the rules and discipline of verbal communication, this is not necessarily the case with the patient.[4]

Interpretations should attempt to capture elements beyond the scope of verbal language. If the language of interpretations articulates these facts, it provides a means to break out of the cycle of projective transformations. These cycles resemble water infiltrating inside a wall, following inefficient paths until a leak becomes visible, with no clear indication of its origin, mirroring the disconnection between meaning and its origin observed in somato-psychotic symptoms or certain maladaptive actions.

An increase in idealization (coinciding with an inhibition of thinking) rather than realization (birth of thoughts) serves as another analogy. However, should communication continue, it enables the discussion and exploration of events at this primitive level of human interaction. This process may initiate a cycle of rigid motion transformations, *during which the past origins of the present situation are elucidated, thereby providing knowledge.* The degree of turbulence associated with hyperboles might seem excluded, yet it constitutes an aspect of non-verbal communication.

5.3   Rigid Motion Transformations

The term "rigid" here does not imply rigidity but refers to the geometric movement of points within space-time. This concept parallels to Freud's use of past events to understand present situations. This understanding, akin to a Freudian interpretation, has the potential to lead to a transformation in knowledge (K). The degree of turbulence is often linked to the mourning of a past object.

5.4   Analytic Transformations in K

This group of transformations focuses on interpretations that facilitate a movement of knowing about oneself (transformations in K) toward a path that may culminate in personal wisdom. However, it is important to recognize that the analyst's role is limited to the point that directs K → (O), marking the *analytic transformation*. The outcome depends entirely on the working through of the analysand; it might or might not lead to transformations in O.

Transformations in O typically transpire outside the analytic field, in a different time-space dimension of the session, possibly manifesting even years after sessions. They happen solely within the analysand's internal time, devoid of any spatial distortion or projection, but rather embody a deep introspection, a "fall" into oneself—not merely knowing about oneself but becoming oneself.

A patient's relationship with themselves can be considered prejudiced if they are unable to advance toward new experiences, reverting instead to familiar meanings. Therefore, a crucial aspect of transformation in O is the acknowledgement of a new experience and the incorporation of new elements.

The next step in this chapter is to illustrate the application of the specific theories outlined by Bion for each type of transformation.

Bion suggests that,

> The analyst's theoretical equipment may thus be narrowly described D4, E4, F4, but the state of mind in which the theories are available in the session should cover a wider spectrum of the grid.[5]

Keeping this provision in mind, he proposes to limit the description of theories to statements falling in the categories E1, E3, E4, and E5. These categories include conceptions or thoughts presented as alternatives, connecting them to the patient's narrative through the evolution of attention that identifies patterns and explores their meanings.

Bion continues, "I mean to employ the following theories:

1 The theory of projective identification and splitting; mechanisms by which the breast provides what the patient later takes over as his own apparatus for α-function.
2 The theory that some personalities cannot tolerate frustration.

3 The theory that a personality with a powerful endowment of envy tends to denude its objects by both stripping and exhaustion.
4 The theory that at an early stage (or on a primitive level of mind) the Oedipal situation is represented by part objects.
5 The Kleinian theory of envy and greed.
6 The theory that primitive thought springs from experience of a non-existing object, or, in other terms, of the place where the object is expected to be, but is not.
7 The theory of violence in primitive functions."[6]

Bion emphasizes that "These theories, as extensions of the Oedipal situation, must be present in the analyst's mind in a form that enables them to be represented in a wide range of grid categories."[7]

I shall now apply these theories to the three basic configurations described by Bion as "commensal, symbiotic, and parasitic,"[8] representing various forms of container/contained relationships. These configurations demarcate the psychoanalytic field for observing catastrophic changes and the corresponding transformations inside the field.

For instance, in *transformations in K*, a harmonious relationship exists between the container and the contained, where theories (6) and (1) are embraced as integral parts of a commensal organization. In other words, the alpha function brings harmony and experience of knowledge between the container and the contained: $(♀)(♂)$.

In *transformations in rigid motion*, a growing disharmony develops between the container and the contained. Therefore, we have theory (1) in conjunction with theory (4), the space of disharmony between the container and the contained is filled with misunderstandings, as extensively elaborated in Freud's theories on transference—elements from the past are perceived as though they belong to the present. At this point, the relationship between the container and the contained, which until now represented a commensal organization, transforms into a symbiotic configuration through the predominance of arrogance.

However, the potential for transition into a symbiotic configuration exists, contingent on the sufficient presence of misunderstandings. Such misunderstandings can lead to numerous mistakes, especially in situations where theory (4) intersects with theory (7).

$$(♀) \text{ Mistakes} + \text{Misunderstandings } (♂)$$

In *projective transformation*, the disharmony between the container and the contained escalates, creating a space that becomes increasingly prone to being permeated with falsehoods. Consequently, additional theories such as (2), (5), (6), and (7) have come into play. This configuration signifies a symbiotic relationship.

$$(♀) \text{ Falsities} + \text{Mistakes} + \text{Misunderstandings } (♂)$$

In *transformation in hallucinosis*, there is an intensification of theory (7), coupled with the highest degree of theory (3), and is further accompanied by theories (5) and (4). Therefore, the discord between the container and the contained escalates to its utmost possible intensity. The space generated by this disharmony becomes saturated with not only lies but also falsities, mistakes, and misunderstandings. This signifies a parasitic configuration.

$$(\female) \text{ Lies} + \text{Falsities} + \text{Mistakes} + \text{Misunderstandings } (\male)$$

Notes

1 W.R. Bion, *Transformations*, 1965, Karnac Books, p. 148.
2 W.R. Bion, *Transformations*, 1965, Karnac Books, p. 78.
3 In *Making the Best of a Bad Job* (1979), Bion outlines *three principles of living:* feelings, anticipatory thinking, and feeling + thinking + Thinking (prudence in action). I believe these are the life values that are attacked when a transformation in hallucinosis develops.
4 W.R. Bion, *Transformations*, 1965, Karnac Books, p. 61.
5 W.R. Bion, *Transformations*, 1965, Karnac Books, p. 51.
6 W.R. Bion, *Transformations*, 1965, Karnac Books, p. 51.
7 W.R. Bion, *Transformations*, 1965, Karnac Books, p. 51.
8 W.R. Bion, *Attention and Interpretation*, 1970, Tavistock. (Re-printed London: Karnac, 1984.)

Chapter 6

Transformations, Time, and Space

Time and space constitute fundamental elements that shape our existence as human beings. Bion's unique conceptualization of space-time within the framework of the theory of transformations represents significant and original contribution to psychoanalysis (Chuster, 1999, 2002, 2014, 2018c, d).

> So far the 'distance' between the analysand's statement (association) and the analyst's statement (interpretation) has been stated in terms of time required for the emergence of the column 2 element in the statement of the analysand and 'proto-resistance,' to coin a phrase, in the analyst to a response that has not yet been made.[1]

Bion recognizes time and space as intrinsic and enduring elements, essential not only to pre-conception but also to conceptions and concepts. This perspective highlights the pivotal role played by the dynamic interplay of time and space in shaping our self-perception as individuals and within the context of social groups.

However, this conceptualization generates a polemic as pre-conception characterized as a vague expectation of a future object that will satisfy all human needs, implying the presence of time in the Unconscious. Nonetheless, this idea is consistent with Bion's investigation of complexity in concepts such as the Act of Faith (1970), Thought Without a Thinker (1970), or his work "A Memoir of the Future" (1975). Exploring this hypothesis, the presence of time in the unconscious, is viable only within the framework of complexity; deterministic or hermeneutic models would fall short in examining such a proposition.

Within the theory of transformations, each type of transformation conveys a distinct *emotional experience* of *time-space* and corresponding *images* (forms) at an unconscious level. These expressions of space-time experiences are basically *unconscious-to-unconscious* communication, a concept alluded to but not explicitly elucidated by Freud.

> The factors that reduce the breast to a point reduce time to 'now'. Time is denuded of past and future. The 'now' is subjected to attacks similar to those delivered against space, or more precisely, the point. It is both exhausted and split.

DOI: 10.4324/9781003474128-7

This leads to expressions which can mislead for such a patient will say 'at the moment' when he means 'never' and 'yesterday' or "tomorrow" when he means a split-off fragment of 'now'; such beliefs contribute to the problems of a patient who cannot tolerate staccato markings in a musical score.[2]

Bion posits that comprehending verbal thoughts through the lens of syntax rules becomes more feasible at an advanced stage of mental development than within the primitive domain he explores. He offers a nuanced, intricate, and profound approach to understanding verbal thoughts in this primitive domain, suggesting the use of basic symbols like the point (.), circle, and line to signify various transformations of emotional experiences of time/space at the deepest layers of unconscious (the raw sensorial level of the mind).

For instance, *transformations in K* generate an experience of time akin to straightforward, logical referential time, linked to a particular image, similar to a point (.) that transforms into a line (————) at more primitive levels of the mind.

In *rigid motion transformations*, the experience of time has a circular nature, reminiscent of a return, paralleling Freud's description of transference. This temporal experience correlates with the image of a circle at more primitive levels of the mind.

The experience of time in *projective transformations* is oscillatory, resembling an undulating movement of a sinusoidal line.

In *Transformations in hallucinosis*, a convergence of various temporal experiences occur, blurring the distinctions between past, present, and future. The unconscious image resembles dispersing lines, akin to a scribble, leading to an emotional experience characterized by confusion and a sense of tyranny.

As we transition from the unconscious depths toward the surface, our perception of time-space undergoes transformation. At the raw sensorial level, we encounter point, circle, sinusoidal line, and scribble. As we progress to more intricate emotional levels, we develop conceptions and, at the experiential level, these conceptions are organized into concepts within the linguistic framework.

The primary challenge involves deciphering the organization of time-space within images across various linguistic levels. The initial meanings of these images reside on the surface of the object. To explore their deeper meanings, one must "scan" the images. This scanning process constitutes the analyst's alpha function, establishing a link between the emitter and the receiver of the images. This link generates a space enriched with connotative symbols, thereby fostering an environment conducive to dreaming and imagination.

It is worth noting that each type of transformation in the analyst corresponds to a form of "scanning" (dreaming, imagination, sensations) of the reality conveyed by the analysand.

For instance, in *transformations in K*, the images establish causal relationships between events, forming a spatial-temporal perception where each segment marks a distinct reference to time, such as "The analytic session is scheduled for 14:00h on Monday." These perceptions closely resemble rational thought, leading to their perception as factual, which may obstruct symbolic interpretations.

In *rigid motion transformations*, a cyclical causality emerges, the past explains the present, which in turn explains the past: (.) ↔ (+). This typically aligns with classical psychoanalytic theory, representing a repetition of past events in the present.

Projective transformations are characterized by what might be termed magical thinking, where the initial idea does not explain the subsequent one, suggesting a disconnect or an absence of meaning in creating a link. For instance, an affirmative like "The rooster's cackle makes the sunrise more beautiful" exhibits + (.) ————, indicating an illogical causality, a transcendence beyond verbal expression, or an absence of meaning.

In *transformations in hallucinosis*, the patient navigates life guided by their subjective images rather than employing images from experiences. This results in a blurred perception of time-space, akin to a disturbing dream or nightmare, where images become ambiguous due to difficulties in transforming them into an abstract dimension. The emergence of these images in the analytic link indicates an analysand who perceives the analyst's interpretations as undermining their logic, evoking feelings of humiliation and prompting retaliatory behaviors to demonstrate the analyst's inadequacy.

To avoid the painful feelings of inferiority, the analysand might adopt a strategy of reversing perspectives, aiming to immobilize the analyst. This reversal of perspectives often evokes familiar states in the analyst, such as drowsiness or a sense of futility in the analysis. Upon interpreting this reversal, if the analysand continues to harbor feelings of superiority, fueled by envy and hatred, the following step involves articulating their attempts to prove the superiority of lies over the search for truth.

Notes

1 W.R. Bion, *Transformations*, 1965, Karnac Books, p. 168.
2 W.R. Bion, *Transformations*, 1965, Karnac Books, p. 55.

Chapter 7

Turbulence and Catastrophic Change

Grasping the concept of Turbulence, rooted in Mathematics and Physics, requires an understanding of complexity theory. For instance, the study of water and air currents, governed by physical laws established nearly two centuries ago, might seem straightforward. However, accurately forecasting the dynamics of these currents during a storm remains impossible. This inherent unpredictability echoes the variable nature of psychoanalytic sessions, where each encounter is distinct.

> There are three features to which I wish to draw attention: subversion of system, invariance and violence.[1]

This unpredictability stems from turbulence, presenting numerous challenges for physicists and mathematicians. Physically, turbulence manifests when a smooth flow of fluid breaks down into smaller eddies and vortices, which then fragment into even finer spirals, generating an unpredictable cascade that disrupts the original smooth flow. These vortices interact in complex ways, rendering the precise prediction of any single particle's behavior impossible. While energy dissipates on a larger scale, presenting an illusion of order, chaos prevails on a smaller scale. Understanding this paradoxical continuous/discontinuous phenomenon is possible only through the lens of complexity theory.

Mathematically, turbulence, initially perceived as straightforward, complicates the application of the Navier–Stokes equations, which have described fluid flows since the early 19th century, accounting for properties like density and viscosity. Although these equations serve well for general predictions, the inherent turbulence in fluids presents a significant challenge, making the consistent application of these equations one of the greatest challenges in physics and mathematics.

The Navier–Stokes equations have proven invaluable in fluid dynamics, with mathematicians striving to ensure that these equations consistently yield meaningful outcomes based on the fluid's initial state. Consider a situation where eddies and vortices concentrate all their energy at a specific point in the fluid, accelerating the flow at that point to an infinite speed. While this scenario is mathematically conceivable yet remains practically unfeasible. This raises a fundamental question: How can we assert the impossibility of an event that has been mathematically validated?

DOI: 10.4324/9781003474128-8

Addressing such a question highlights the inherent complexity we must face, requiring the exercise of patience and a stance of *negative capability*—awaiting the future while actively participating in it. A notable illustration of this complexity is evident in ideas spanning centuries, maintaining vitality, and evolving into new versions.

The question explores the capacity of the *social body* to establish links with the ideas of mystics/geniuses and, ultimately, either contain or nurture them. It revolves around the *observer*. This dialogue aims to draw parallels and distinctions between mystics/geniuses and the social body, offering insights that may prove valuable in analytic practice. It examines how psychoanalysts, in clinical settings, approach the role of a "mystic/genius," perceiving and interpreting complex facts not readily expressible by common language, yet offering practical insights for patients' personal growth.

In practice, psychoanalysts serve as anonymous interpreters of diverse perceptions of no lesser literary and artistic value. Within the anonymity of potent ideas emerging in the humble context of an analyst/analysand relationship, interpretations engage with the unconscious, aiming to demystify the mystic and unseat the genius. Following the Latin adage "*Sapere Aude*" (dare to know), this approach emphasizes resisting any psychoanalytic authority that seeks to inhibit our thoughts.

Culture establishes the links between the social body and individuals characterized by mystical and genius qualities. In this context, culture functions as a *caesura* between the mystic/genius and the group. Mystics and geniuses emerge from within the group, yet simultaneously distinguish themselves from the group by surpassing common sense. In the discussions that follow, I will explore psychoanalytic culture and its interplay with the essence of a never-ending psychoanalytic revolution.

The facts presented aim to examine a favorable or opposing stance toward the ideas articulated by mystics or geniuses. From this perspective, we can investigate specific cultures that exhibit the confusion between science and religion, as well as the politicization or publication of these ideas.

Certain religious cultures advocate for the exclusion, and in some cases, the destruction of art. Additionally, certain highly rigid religious cultures exclusively endorse domesticated forms of art and prohibit any engagement with cultures that politicize science.

Encountering Freud's work necessitates a discussion on the ideas proposed by mystics or geniuses. Bion begins this discourse toward the end of *Transformations* (1965) and further elaborates on them further in *Attention and Interpretation* (1970).

Plato once advocated for the exclusion of poetry from education, a notion that has endured in contemporary educational practices. He posited that poetry could corrupt the minds of youth. This stance gave rise to *didacticism*, founded on the belief that city walls could educate the citizens; similarly, invisible institutional walls were thought to elevate the quality of education. Didacticism gave rise to *Conservatism*, characterized by maintaining a fixed curriculum, which eventually led to the development of *Romanticism* and educational ideals that proved unattainable. The impossibility of these ideals resulted in the emergence of an administrative class known as the governing elite or *Establishment*, wherein priests could hold prominent roles.

For instance, during Newton's era, the Bishop of Berkeley "attacked certain illogicalities, notably circular argument, in Newton's presentation of the differential calculus; his criticisms exercised mathematicians for over a century."[2] This illustrates how conservatism and a blind Platonic didactic approach attack creativity.

Newton's formulation of differential calculus represents a transformation in knowledge (K), despite being based on ideas his contemporaries deemed psychotic, such as "the ghosts of departed quantities."

Fortunately, Plato conveyed Socrates' wisdom, who conducted his teachings outside the city walls and emphasized the importance of acquiring proficiency in poetry as a crucial aspect of an individual's education. Socrates likened himself to a midwife, assisting in the birth of ideas. Hence, even in contemporary times, genuine learning requires stepping outside the confines of walls and engaging in discussions about ideas. This movement must be both continuous and discontinuous, involving transitions from inside to outside and vice versa.

Notes

1 W.R. Bion, *Transformations*, 1965, Karnac Books, p. 8.
2 W.R. Bion, *Transformations*, 1965, Karnac Books, p. 157.

Chapter 8

Catastrophic Change and Cultural Possibilities

The possibilities for cultural expressions are infinite and always implicated in transformations. Bion's (1965, 1970) perspectives provide us with tools to observe symmetries across the three principal human activities—science, art, and religion. These symmetries stem from *Oedipal configurations* identified as *commensal*, *symbiotic*, and *parasitic*. These configurations denote three general types of culture and distinct container/contained relationships that influence human activities.

> In my illustration it is possible that we shall need to discuss the lay point of view, such as that involved in concluding that the patient is not simply a normal person being difficult, but that he is mentally disturbed.[1]

Every culture inherently embodies distinct practices governed by a system and a complex set of explicit and implicit relations of meanings that manifest in the realms of thought, action, and emotion. In essence, there exists a continuous dynamic cycle that interrelates emotional experiences, actions, and the ongoing creation of knowledge.

The apex of emotional experiences in Bion follows Freud's view of the Oedipus myth as a gateway to culture, serving as a heuristic tool for investigation. In essence, the Oedipal configuration plays a determining role in an individual's thinking, acting, and feeling within a culture. Alternatively, culture is an amalgamation of interactions among individuals who adopt common patterns of thinking and behavior to foster unity.

The transition from one Oedipal configuration to another is an example of *catastrophic change*. This term is often misunderstood as a *disaster* or *calamity* within certain psychoanalytic circles. However, this change is not a disaster; rather, it reflects the profound meaning embedded in the Greek tragedy of Oedipus. This tragedy has served as a catalyst for explorations into the unconscious, such as those undertaken by Freud in the development of psychoanalysis. The Oedipal tragedy stands as an unparalleled exemplar, epitomizing how we think, imagine, dream, and represent our perceptions of parents, riddles, knowledge, power, the environment, and, essentially, every aspect that shapes human culture. Above all, while

DOI: 10.4324/9781003474128-9

one navigates this course, the journey unfolds as a perpetual process of discovering and rediscovering psychoanalysis.

A natural catastrophe, like an earthquake, compels us to confront the remains of what once existed, within the context of its former configuration. In a psychoanalytic context, understanding the post-catastrophic states cannot be approached with a notion of *truth-suitability*,[2] as one might in the case of a natural disaster. We cannot simply dismiss the facts of the pre-catastrophic states as mere historical past, nor as a linear logic; rather, we should use non-linear logics to incorporate them into a truthful expression of outcomes. In other words, dialogical thinking is required to develop observations of new and unknown facts.

Freud's[3] assertion regarding the continuity between intra-uterine life and earliest infancy might be paraphrased, as "there is much more continuity between one person and another, between one configuration and another." This assertion encourages us to focus on examining the observer who strives to perceive facts as they are, acknowledging their interference (the observer transforming the observed) and accepting the inherent incompleteness in situations where nothing can be fully understood or resolved.

I acknowledge the challenge inherent in a debate between these two "truths," the observer and the observed. Turbulence is an ever-present element that intensifies upon closer examination. Consequently, instead of adhering to a dialectical approach, I favor the concept of *complexity*.

Complexity liberates us from the restrictive coercion of dialectics. Dialectical methods often lead to a false sense of resolution by simplistically accepting that in every case, both similarities and differences must be acknowledged. This approach, characterized by simplistic and positivistic generalizations, has led to the phenomenon currently known as "politically correct speech."

To be politically correct, one is often expected to eliminate certain expressions from their vocabulary to respect differences and promote equality for all. However, since true equality can only be achieved through ethical means, we may find ourselves pretending that there are no differences, despite being aware of their persistent reality. In this endeavor, we might convince ourselves of our righteousness, contributing to social harmony, while labeling those who diverge from these norms as wrong. This represents a form of moralistic thinking that masks dictatorial tendencies and is closely linked to *hypocrisy*, forming the "-H" link in Bion's framework.

In this context, one might apply a phrase often attributed to Nietzsche: *The Elite is constantly inventing habits and words in which it ends up believing.*[4]

The scope of hypocrisy (-H) throughout human history appears boundless. One example of this is the adoption of models from other cultures, frequently considered superior to those of the original culture. This phenomenon can be termed *cultural provincialism* at its least. It represents a significant contemporary dilemma when individuals reject their own culture in favor of something unfamiliar, lacking any personal emotional experience. From a detached viewpoint, motivated by envy and other emotions arising from an inability to create, one might mistakenly believe that the grass is greener on the other side.

In the realm of Oedipus, pacification appears elusive—a constant turbulence inherent in the human condition. Freud's contributions signified a major paradigm shift. Bion's spectrum model explores infinite possibilities, expanding Freud's ideas and introducing numerous semantic innovations and a novel worldview, leading to a fresh understanding of the self. The forthcoming ideas try to elucidate these possibilities.

Bion's (1970) analysis of the language of mystics reveals that it would be erroneous to regard it as purely poetic. While it undeniably contains poetic elements characterized by an abundance of wild thoughts, Bion also highlights that the concept of "O," which mystics refer to as "God," is subtly present in Milton's works.

Milton alluded to the *void* and *formless infinite*. Kant described it as the "thing in itself," a scientist might call it an *ultimate reality*, and an artist may consider it an *absolute reality*. These interpretations align with Buber's depiction, as mentioned by Bion,[5] that a man in his mother's womb knows the universe and forgets it at birth. The question remains: what is this forgotten reality?

Mystics and geniuses are those who, unlike most, do not forget this primitive hidden reality. Melanie Klein, for instance, appears to have maintained vivid memories of infancy, as reflected in her extensive theory. Winnicott vividly recalled moments from his early childhood, such as playing with a pillow. Einstein, inspired by his childhood imagination of riding a beam of light through the universe, later translated this idea into an unprecedented and groundbreaking contribution to physics as an adult.

Every literary form, ranging from narratives and folktales to poetry and fiction, represents evolutions of "O." This perspective does not contradict the inherent qualities of poems, regardless of whether they are perceived as text, art, or science. Bion goes beyond narratives and speeches while focusing on "O."

The concept of "O" suggests a continuous circulation, an ongoing development of an original *ideogram*. This ideogram simultaneously generates the texts and remains elusive to them. Investigating how "O" manifests in text, speech, or other human expressions can be accomplished through the mutation of meaning. Identifying this meaning is crucial for outlining the nature of transformation, as Bion discussed in *Transformations* (1965).

It is tempting to associate this mutation of meaning solely with what could be termed "limit-expressions."[6] Such expressions include the unknowable, the absolute Truth, the original preconception, the trance, and the elements of psychoanalysis. While Bion's employment of these limit-expressions certainly emphasizes the specificity of language, they do not entirely define it. Words, as carriers of thoughts and emotions, function within the framework of an essentially metaphorical analog language, embodied by the descriptive, prescriptive, prophetic, and, ultimately, parabolic nature of "O." These *limit-expressions* serve to qualify, modify, and rectify this analog language, paving the way for the digital, symbolic language.

On the other hand, artistic narratives, religious prophecies, and scientific laws operate not merely at the conceptual level but at the level of *diagrams*. Drawing from Kant's notion of schema,[7] it represents "a universal procedure of imagination in providing an image for a concept," not just to an idea, or even the *Idea*, as outlined in the Theory of Aesthetic Ideas, but rather to what Kant qualifies as essence. Epistemologically, schemata are rules that govern the production of figures like the priest, scientist, artist, judge, father, husband, mother, servant, and others.

These figures are not just pure expressions of "O" undergoing transformation; they are articulated to adapt a specific group to a particular culture. This accounts for their enduring diversity, heterogeneity, and inability to form a standalone system. Moreover, no approach is devoid of a conceptual foundation. This is why the predominant trend in representing the idol is anthropomorphic, exemplified in science by the genius, in art by the charismatic artist, and in religion by the mystic. In clinical practice, this equates to placing trust in the patient's appearance or job title and believing in their authority on a specific subject.

For instance, consider a scenario where a man, dressed in the formal attire of a Federal Supreme Court judge, enters our office. It presents a potential risk to assume maturity, erudition, and expertise based solely on his attire. Indeed, by not being misled by this conceptual anthropomorphic image, we might gain insight (when relevant analytic material arises) into why this apparently mature individual might suddenly display fury, akin to a young boy feeling aggrieved because his mother had a new baby, when the psychoanalyst takes on a new patient.

In another scenario, we might meet a successful medical doctor who expresses concerns about feeling unsafe in his office. Through analysis, could we uncover motivations such as a hidden desire to harm people or a sense of frustration stemming from unfulfilled hero complex expectations?

The psychoanalyst consistently strives to avoid conceptual pitfalls that could lead to *the idealization of models*. To address these challenges, I propose substituting the conventional dialectic model with an *ethics of complex thinking*. This entails discarding fixed personalization and reinstating "O" as a domain. In doing so, we can examine how "O" governs the schema within the current models employed by the patient—creating, influencing, energizing, and disseminating it, akin to the dynamics in the Oedipus myth as represented by the family group characters. This method adopts a dialogic model, promoting a more nuanced understanding of the complexities inherent in the patient's psyche.

"O" manifests as Oedipus, Laius, or Jocasta, and simultaneously embodies all of these entities. Bion's dialogic approach advocates for the use of all characters and passages from Sophocles' three plays, thus expanding the scope of the myth. Further delving into other myths, such as those of Eden, Babel, excerpts from the Aeneid, the construction of facts through assumptions in archaeological discoveries, and the myth of Prometheus, can enrich the poietic-psychoanalytic discourse. The possibilities are infinite, especially when aligned with the emotional turbulence vividly portrayed in these myths. This extensive exploration augments the depth of the psychoanalytic inquiry.

Dialogic thinking adheres to Kant's *Idea*, necessitating the transcendence not only of the *image* but also of the *concept* by encouraging us to "think more." With "O" as a primary reference, dialogic thinking challenges all models while simultaneously deriving strength from them.

In correlating "O" with the cultural idol, which signifies the schema interpreted by mystics or geniuses, we uncover the significant role of Bion's theory concerning *limit-expressions*.

A prime example of utilizing limit-expressions is Bion's Grid, which serves as a tool for the *functional analysis* of an action and its retrospective impact in generating future outcomes. Essentially, *a posteriori* critique within the Grid forms hypotheses for future application. The Grid, as a vectorial space comprised entirely of limit-expressions, strives to be a transformative instrument for the interpretive models used in psychoanalysis.

By employing Bion's Grid for reflective thinking after sessions, we can circumvent a reductive approach to language, such as the simplistic conversion of poetic language into religious language. It is essential to recognize that figures like Milton, who seemingly engaged in such transitions, did so with a level of complexity. In Milton's "Paradise Lost," the apparent shift from poetic to religious language masks a profound political critique of his era. This underscores the importance of acknowledging the intricate layers and nuanced dimensions in language and its transformations.

A consistent presence of models that generate transformations in knowledge (K) is noted. However, these models may introduce paradoxes, leading to types of catastrophic changes, such as transformations in rigid motion. When knowledge assumes a hyperbolic dimension, it results in the creation of projective transformations. Similarly, the emergence of negative or mind-destructive meanings can lead to changes, exemplified by lies acting as catalysts for transformations in hallucinosis. This complex interplay highlights the intricacies and potential ramifications inherent in the evolution of transformations within the realm of K.

The domain of poetics intrinsically incorporates an aspect of "rebuilding" or "repairing" the world, as conceptualized in Klein's terminology. This process of reconstruction is steered by a distinctive "vertex" that is inherent to the poem or metaphor. Within this context, employing Klein's hermeneutical approach signifies a crucial point of understanding.

Bion's dialogic model introduces an alternative approach to language, one that fundamentally incorporates *uncertainty* and *indeterminism*. This perspective shifts the emphasis from acquiring knowledge to self-transformation. Such language bypasses the conventional paths of intellect or common sense. Bion's methodology surpasses mere hermeneutics; it embodies the realization of words as "public-action" (1970), signifying *indetermination.* In this context, exploring and transforming one's inner world are essentially unified processes.

In Klein's framework, the strength and logic of limit-expressions acquire a deeply symbolic significance, echoing the philosophical style of Kierkegaard. However, in Bion's dialogical model, these limit-expressions do not dictate any specific conduct. This approach necessitates exercising psychoanalysis at the heart of emotional experience, requiring a suspension of memory, desire, and the need for comprehension, thus promoting *interpretative symmetry* where life's *limit-experiences* constantly meet.

Despite a superficial congruence between *limit-experiences* and *limit-expressions*, Bion views these as precursors to inevitable catastrophic changes. This process involves navigating through ethics and public-action to achieve a positive, though unstable and temporary role in analogous "models" (interpretations that encompass everything the analyst experiences in the session, transforming him into an excavator of transference rather than a mere supportive operator). This transcendence is based on the concept of *negative capability* (Bion, 1970), similar to Keats's focus on the poet's mental attitude over the poetry itself, a principle that is equally relevant for psychoanalysts.

Understanding the key difference in Bion's dialogical model is vital, particularly its emphasis on ethics in *public-action* (1970) as a guiding principle for humanity. Psychoanalytic language, through symmetrical analytical constructions, aims to free humanity. This involves, for example, not discussing omnipotence without helplessness.

Meltzer (1996) recognized Bion's humanistic approach. However, it is crucial to differentiate this orientation from demagogic rhetoric or adherence to politically correct standards. Various elements of culture, including language resources, myths, and dreams, serve as tools enabling us to appreciate the humanism in the Oedipal mind without falling prey to hidden ideological influences on our modes of action, thought, or feeling. When such influences become apparent, a psychoanalytic deception satisfies the analyst's romantic notions and indulges their hallucinatory pleasure.

Models stemming from the Oedipus myth, which might also encompass myths like Babel, Eden, the death of Palinurus, Prometheus, Medea, Antigone, among others, are essentially poetic rather than political.

The discourse on symbiotic culture often confronts scenarios where "culture" is used as a catch-all term for various practices, many of which lack genuine belief or conviction. These practices, though not always taken earnestly, carry an emotional experience that can confer true value on them. The nature of a symbiotic configuration is that the connection between its elements is defined by opposing forces, similar to a "tug of war."

Santa Claus is an exemplary case of these contradictory forces. While Christian adults may not believe in him, they encourage their children to eagerly await the mythical Santa Claus, creating a euphoric reality. They justify this joyous illusion as part of "lifestyle," maintaining a "tradition." This cultural approach often overlooks the potential disillusionment and distress a child might feel upon discovering the truth behind the myth. Could this realization affect the child's future perception of reality and their trust in parents and authority figures?

Diminished trust in what was once a commensal family relationship can lead to a catastrophic change. The child might eventually believe that their parents are capable of deceit and that dishonesty is embedded in the culture. This realization could relate to both minor and more serious issues, such as sexual abuse, bullying, or drug use, potentially causing the child to harbor secrets and hesitate to share certain experiences with their parents.

In this scenario, a traditional family might be characterized as one that engages in actions contradicting its beliefs, leading its members to experience this hypocrisy. Hypocrisy in this context could be conceptualized as the -H link, fostering an ideal environment for the cultivation of hate.

Following this trajectory, it becomes evident that concepts of style and tradition are rooted in the creation and perpetuation of lies, possibly driven by the sheer pleasure that manifests in consumerism.

This notion leads to the presumption that anyone who diverges from the established style or tradition is erroneous or misguided. Those who criticize this hypocrisy are often labeled as "killjoys," while those who object based on the principle of reality are frequently deemed "boring."

The maxim, "Seek pleasure at all costs, damn reality," or its variant, "Live for the moment," highlights immediate gratification, signifying a distinct moral position steeped in unbridled hedonism. Exploring the range of morals arising from these covert representations might yield significant insights. For example, Santa Claus, symbolizing Jesus/God during Christmas, represents a morality focused on self-sacrifice for children's happiness, embodying sacrificial morality.

The characteristics of catastrophic change become evident when the container/ contained relationship transitions from symbiotic to parasitic are exemplified in the application of science in cultures with limited capacity for critical thought. In such environments, science often clashes with deep-seated traditions that demand adherence to established beliefs. Therefore, where beliefs overshadow reality, the importance of factual reality diminishes. For example, fundamentalists typically dismiss scientific views. Yet, in their communities, more moderate religious figures sometimes advocate for science. Occasionally, a scientific concept may transform into a belief, where truth is swayed by momentary convenience, becoming a cultural endeavor for truth-suitability, aligning truth with cultural beliefs.

For instance, fundamentalists reject Darwin's theory of evolution. They struggle to interpret the Bible as a poetic and metaphorical text. Many believe that the Bible is more "scientific" than Darwin's work. From the perspective of fundamentalism, the scientist is merely a purveyor of a significant falsehood. The parasitic relationship that undermines Darwin's scientific notions arises from the fundamentalist belief that the world is as described in the Bible, having begun exactly 5780 years ago, as stated in the scripture.

Indeed, this scenario exemplifies a logical fallacy. The argument that defines a term (or concept) using the term itself for justification is inherently circular. An example of this is the assertion: "The Bible is the Word of God because it states that it is the Word of God." To substantiate the claim of the Bible's divine origin, the Bible itself is evidence. This is a circular argument.

If there is concrete archaeological evidence, backed by rigorous scientific research, showing that species existed millions of years ago, fundamentalists might dismiss this as a fabrication by atheists to undermine religion. It is important to acknowledge that the persistence of this *parasitic* viewpoint is a result of its continuous reinforcement within a specific cultural context.

If these fundamentalists existed in isolation, they would likely find harmony and commonality within their group. However, in a culture where the majority are not fundamentalists, a symbiotic cultural dynamic could still be present. In such a case, one group might attempt to dominate or neutralize the other driven by primitive group mechanisms.

Assuming the vertex of a culture's integrity of ideas involves embracing various viewpoints seriously, without adopting a critical stance. Fundamentalists, who interpret the Bible literally cannot perceive its text metaphorically. Conversely, those who regard science as paramount might see believers as obstructive, labeling them "barbarians" or "uncivilized" and accusing them of impeding human progress—a clear allegation of *parasitism*. Yet, fundamentalists firmly hold onto their beliefs, which others dismiss as fantasy. This leads to the question: What distinguishes these groups if both are intolerant of opposing views?

This secular hypocrisy arises from a lack of critical detachment. A scientist who overlooks the need for critical distance in scientific inquiry is as problematic as fundamentalists are. However, what are the consequences of this lack of critical distance? For instance, many self-identified Catholics neither regularly attend church nor believe in Jesus. Yet, when it suits them, they participate in church rituals and might even blame Jews for the crucifixion of Christ.

This pattern of hypocrisy and hatred is pervasive across religions and extends into politics. Political parties often condone corruption, rationalizing it as a part of political culture, and quickly denounce their critics as fascists. A behavior often seen in Leninists or left-wing extremists is accusing and blaming their opponents for the very actions and traits they themselves display. This kind of thinking reflects in the spectrum covered by the H and -H (hypocrisy) links.

Fascists and Nazis took their ideologies with utmost seriousness. The inquisitors, arguably more than any other group, can be seen as their direct ancestors. These groups share notable similarities, particularly in their prioritization of the State above all. They effectively deified the State. Within this cultural framework, individuals routinely speak as if they are representatives of the State. Fascist newspapers, adhering to this doctrine, act as mouthpieces for the State.

Both the Fascists and Nazis obscured the line between the State and the government. The Nazis rapidly co-opted science to bolster their political ideology, using it to justify genocidal actions. Concentration camps, influenced by genetic science, were designed to assess genetic fitness for survival. While termed concentration camps, their primary function was extermination, operating like factories of death. The language used to describe them was deeply hypocritical. These instances vividly demonstrate that when beliefs override critical thinking, the importance of reality diminishes.

When General Eisenhower became aware of the numerous concentration camps, he ordered extensive filming of the atrocities, anticipating future denials. His experience in combating dictators had sharpened his intuition about transformations in hallucinosis, which promote rigid mental processes rooted in exclusive beliefs and dogmas, often advanced by dictators. His foresight also recognized humanity's historical inclination to deny genocides, leading him to take preemptive action.

The inquisitors, a major historical influence on the cruelty of Nazis and Fascists, have never completely vanished; they often manifest today in contemporary newspapers as a kind of ideological guard. This guard, rooted in political control by the State, has agents ready to intrude in Education, Art, Justice, and Science. Their goal is to foster a culture of uniformity, systematically eradicating any form of difference.

The primary objective of the Inquisition was indeed to fabricate alibis that would enable embezzlement and corruption. This pattern of behavior repeated in the actions of the Nazis, who were adept at looting treasures from the people they dominated. In the extermination camps, they achieved a level of cruel sophistication by extracting gold fillings from their victims to forge ingots, which sustained their war efforts. This ideology, it appears, has a persistent and enduring presence. This war never ends, that is, obtaining cultural success by erasing the stains from the megalomaniac narcissistic painting of purity.

Notes

1 W.R. Bion, *Transformations*, 1965, Karnac Books, p. 10.
2 Muniz Sodré, *A Verdade Seduzida*, 1988, Francisco Alves. *Truth-suitability*, as a philosophical concept used by Sodré, involves attempting to compel truth to conform to specific, often agreeable patterns.
3 S. Freud, "There is much more continuity between intra-uterine life and earliest infancy than the impressive caesura of the act of birth would have us believe." *Inhibitions, Symptoms and Anxiety*, 1926, SE Vol. XX, p. 138.
4 F. Nietzsche, *Beyond Good and Evil: Prelude to a Philosophy of the Future*, first published in 1886.
5 W.R. Bion, *The Complete Works of W. R. Bion*, 2014, edited by Chris Mawson, Vol. X, pp. 35–36.
6 Limit-expressions, as an epistemological concept, denote the maximal abstraction achievable in expression, beyond which meaning is lost.
7 Immanuel Kant, *Critique of Pure Reason*, translated by Norman Kemp Smith, 2007, Palgrave Macmillan, pp. 182–183. Editor's note, Kant differentiates between schema and image. Schema is "a product and, as it were, a monogram, of pure *a priori* imagination, through which, and in accordance with which, images themselves first become possible. These images can be connected with the concept only by means of the schema to which they belong.... The concept 'dog' signifies a rule according to which my imagination can delineate the figure of a four-footed animal in a general manner, without limitation to any single, determinate figure, such as experience, or any possible image that I can represent *in concreto*, actually presents" (p. 183).

Chapter 9

Exploring Complexity

Functions of the Psychoanalytic Object in Analysis

An epistemological approach is essential in this context. It could be described as the "*object of psychoanalysis*," conceptualized as the culmination of an author's theoretical and clinical development. This framework, instrumental in evaluating interventions and interpretations within the analytical process, must be dynamic. It should include mechanisms that not only facilitate the evolution of ideas but also prioritize the observation of facts that are subject to transformations.

> I had hoped to write this book so that it could be read independently of Learning from Experience and Elements of psychoanalysis, but I soon found this impossible without an intolerable degree of repetition.[1]

> The term 'transformation' may mislead unless the limitations of the implication of 'form' are recognized.[2]

For Bion, the object of psychoanalysis is the "*psychoanalytic object*" (1962b), corresponding to Freud's concept of superego, Melanie Klein's internal objects, Winnicott's transitional object, Lacan's real/symbolic/imaginary ties, and Green's central phobic position.

The object of psychoanalysis holds paradigmatic significance. Therefore, it is imperative to explore its extent of influence on the methodology, logic, epistemology, ontology, and, most critically, on the analyst's practice.

This chapter will not delve into the object of psychoanalysis as interpreted by other authors; instead, it will concentrate on Bion, aiming to trace the sequence of inquiries that unfold throughout his texts.

In *Learning from Experience*,[3] Bion introduces the formula of the psychoanalytic object employing mathematical-like characters:

$$\left\{ \psi\left(\xi\right)\left(\pm Y\right)\mu \right\}$$

DOI: 10.4324/9781003474128-10

This mathematical formulation may be unfamiliar to many analysts. Nonetheless, it aligns with Bion's *Theory of Thinking* (1962a), where he intuitively employs a complex mode of thought, positioning psychoanalysis at the intersection of mathematics and philosophy. A brief review of this theory is warranted before proceeding.

The "*Theory of Thinking*" (Bion, 1962a) proposes that psychoanalysis serves as a practical response to philosophical inquiries—those life questions for which philosophers possess an enhanced capacity for theoretical elaboration but lack practical-poietic activity. However, for psychoanalysis to effectively link with philosophy, it must emulate the same link between pure and applied mathematics. This necessitates that psychoanalysis delineates its domain to ascertain its boundaries and possibilities. Crucially, it must identify the epistemological principles governing its field to avoid empty habits, trivial repetitions, and commonplace beliefs, thereby fostering the emergence of novel questions and *wild* thoughts.

The psychoanalyst is not a philosopher or a mathematician, despite any aspirations to be one. Nevertheless, psychoanalytic practice necessitates a receptivity to mathematical and philosophical elements for the development of thinking. This receptivity hinges on epistemological principles that safeguard the use of intuition and imagination in clinical practice. These *ethical-aesthetical principles* have been described in various publications. Notably, the Uncertainty Principle, a cornerstone of the Theory of Complexity, appears particularly pertinent for initiating discussion.

Complexity, a constellation of various ideas, elucidates numerous "enigmatic" concepts of Bion, with the psychoanalytic object being one of the most illustrative (Chuster, 2014, 2018, 2020). Essentially, the psychoanalytic object signifies the transition from the *simple object* to the *complex object* in psychoanalysis. Understanding these concepts can be challenging, especially when juxtaposed with other psychoanalytic models. While these models remain valuable, it is crucial to set them aside, without drawing comparisons, to fully grasp Bion's endeavor in developing a new model of thinking.[4]

In a field governed by epistemological principles, the mathematical requirement primarily suggests a mode of thinking aimed at avoiding saturation with meanings. This process begins with writing at a high level of abstraction. The essence of analytical work lies in the discovery of meaning. There is no *a priori* for the meaning of the psychoanalytic object. Meanings may or may not emerge during the analytical work.

Bion's formula can be translated as follows: *pre-conception* ψ (ξ) seeks a *Realization* (R) and gives birth to a *conception* within the spectrum ($\pm Y$). This spectrum extends from the $-Y$ (minus *Why?*) pole (narcissism) to the $+Y$ (plus *Why?*) pole (social-ism), under the constant aegis of *complexity* (μ mystery), a characteristic fundamental to all biological organisms (Chuster, 1999, 2002, 2018b). Figure 9.1 attempts to illustrate the multidimensional aspect of my description:

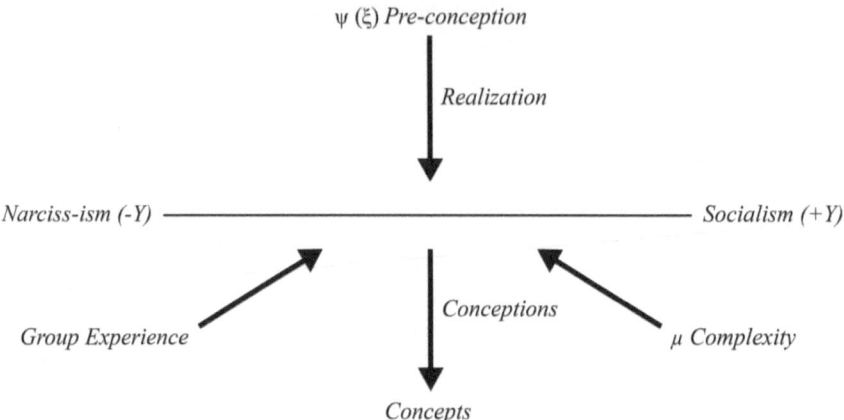

Figure 9.1 Psychoanalytic Object.

In elaborating on these concepts, it can be stated that the initial stage of a pre-conception's realization in its search for a conception invariably transpires through conceptions/beliefs. This is due to the crude emotions and the influence of external reality—not-me—from which the experience appears to originate.

Suppose these conceptions develop narcissistic tendencies (-Y) within the spectrum, caused by the alpha function's failure to process the emotional impact of a pre-conception. At this moment of a not-me experience, the conceptions may solidify into firm beliefs and dogmas. This can lead to significant difficulty, or even an impossibility (due to heavy saturation with meanings), in progressing to the level of *thinking*. From the thinking level, it becomes feasible to advance to the level of *learning from experience*, and subsequently to the level of *creation*, which can introduce novel and singular elements. The creation level, in turn, initiates a complex interplay with numerous variables, forming a loop in search of pre-conceptions (origins).

In a fundamentalist society, dogmas (hyper-saturated knowledge) imprison individuals within fierce narcissistic spheres, markedly limiting or altogether negating possibilities for creation. In such societies, artistic fields are virtually non-existent. Beliefs stifle the capacity for thinking and inhibit creativity. In other words, beliefs and dogmas are conceptions and concepts that lose the value of pre-conception—the very root that facilitates the genesis of new conceptions.[5]

The deprivation of thinking activity, encompassing the capacity for doubt—and the doubt of doubt itself—compromises the attainment of creativity and freedom, thereby undermining the potential for respecting life. Chuster (2018d, 2020) identifies respect for life and truth as components of an analytical ethical barrier, likening it to a psychoanalyst's guardian angel.

The alpha function is responsible for facilitating contact and negotiation between inner and outer realities. Metaphorically, it serves to digest or filter sensory impressions of raw reality and intense emotions, thus enabling the psychic apparatus to contain and utilize them.

Psychological growth fundamentally involves tolerance and coping with failures and frustrations. Meltzer (1996) posits the existence of two types of alpha function. The first, the alpha function of the Self, serves as a container for meanings emanating from external reality and is inherently incomplete, as it must embody a certain degree of failure. This aligns with a dream model; one may conjecture that if an individual experienced a perfect dream, there would be no impetus to awaken. Moreover, it is through the dream's failure that awareness of the body and awakening occur. The second type pertains to the alpha function of internal objects.

The inevitable failure of alpha function can find support by two mental functions: the intuitive and the social. A developed intuitive function can evolve into mystical ideas, science, art, or the psychoanalytic function of the personality. The analytic work[6] can be the training for the latter.

The social function helps the individual in addressing facts and situations that are beyond their capacity to manage alone. These encompass laws, rituals, codes, ceremonies, and similar elements. The social function is fundamentally historical, providing references that enable the individual's historical context to locate itself within the group identity. In general, conceptions and concepts intrinsically incorporate their own alpha function, which enhances the containing capacity of the psychoanalytic object.

The concept of Realization, which represents the most intricate aspect of the psychoanalytic object, is often simplistically perceived as merely the process of saturation by reality. That is, the notion that once a preconception encounters reality, it yields a conception. This oversimplification arises because psychoanalytic literature overlooks the fact that Realization is a mathematical tool (Chuster, 1999, 2002, 2014, 2018, 2020).

By highlighting the mathematical foundation of the concept of Realization and incorporating the epistemology of Complexity, a distinct perspective for investigating the process of Realization emerges. Approaching from this novel vertex of inquiry, it becomes evident that Realization is not merely a simple grammatical term signifying the achievement of something. Rather, it is a concept applicable when a paradigm shift toward complexity is required, as expounded by Bion in his *Theory of Thinking* (1962a).

The origins of this shift can be traced back to when Bion distinguished himself from other Kleinian authors through identifying the mechanism of projective identification as the primary process of communication, rather than merely defining it as an unconscious phantasy.

Projective identification, the fundamental process of communication—or the most primitive social form of human connection—is a continuous unconscious psychic movement that ceases only upon reaching its targeted object. Operating at an unconscious level, it surmounts all barriers, manifesting its impact through the emotional states that surface across various levels of human experience. This phenomenon underpins the origin of Bion's ideas regarding the emergence and development of emotional experience.

Freud's model of the mind has the theory of repression as one of its core concepts. Repression can be envisioned as a barrier that disrupts the drives, leading them to partially revert onto themselves. Within this model, the partial overcoming of the repression barrier creates the exteriorization of the unconscious (such as symptom formation) and contributes to the formation of the so-called "Unconscious." The prevailing paradigm of this theory is the compulsion to repetition. Interpretations of the analytic field typically link repetitions of past events to present meanings. These interpretations align with Bion's concept of transformations in rigid motion (1965).

In Bion's model, exteriorization transpires through *conceptions* and their capacity (or lack thereof) to retain the value of pre-conception. When a conception maintains the value of a pre-conception, it has the potential to generate new conceptions (+Y). Conversely, a decrease in this value gives rise to beliefs. When conceptions establish a *constant conjunction*,[7] they gain the capacity to turn into concepts, forging links between our internal world and that of others. This evolution of conceptions to concepts is attributed to the group experience.

It could be posited that an expansion paradigm, encompassing evolution and restoration, governs the field delineated by Bion. Interpretations typically aim to connect intuitive perception, imaginative creation, and transformation. The essence of creativity hinges on a background of discipline (negative capability), highlighting the importance of remaining receptive to second thoughts.

Bion's *Theory of Thinking* (1962a) introduced a paradigm shift with epistemological inquiries related to a new theory of the Unconscious, aspects of which are not always explicit. In addition, as noted in the introduction, this shift requires acknowledging the epistemological distinctions in the methodology of observation, the logic of the theory, its ontology, and, ultimately, the implications of these in practice.

The insights into the alterations wrought by the emotional experience of human being in their ceaseless quest for psychic objects illuminate how Bion discusses the transition from pre-human to human, among various topics (Chuster, 2014, 2018, 2020). This transition highlights an eternal *inaccessibility* to this human origin, which Bion (1965) referred to as "O."

Due to this inaccessibility, Bion proposes the existence of three mental states: *inaccessible* ↔ *unconscious* ↔ *conscious*. Subsequently, he suggests its replacement by the spectrum infinite ↔ finite. The latter version can be further developed into a proposition of a *Principle of Infinitude*[8] within the analytical field (Chuster 1997c, d).

The *principle of infinitude* in Bion's ideas proposes a perpetual expansion of the unconscious, owing to the extension of the knowledge (K) link, which serves as a conductor for emotional experience. As the K link introduces elements of uncertainty and incompleteness, the growth (evolution) of the mind takes place simultaneously with reparation. The complexity inherent in these concurrent movements offers a means to observe and explore the mystery of the mind.

A practical application of this concept views every word in the communication process (public-action) as perpetually open to *infinite* realities. This perspective can also be juxtaposed with the ideas expressed in the concept of the *act-of-faith* (Bion, 1970), a term borrowed from Nietzsche.[9] It is important to note that this term does not relate to faith as a belief, but rather to creation.

The theory of pre-conception, serving as the ontological foundation of the psychoanalytic object raises numerous scientific, philosophical, and epistemological questions that extend beyond Bion's era. While Bion did not explicitly articulate these questions, he engaged with them intuitively, demonstrating both resourcefulness and courage. This approach can be seen as a Memoir of the Future.

Bion's ontological approach encompasses the element of preconception, which is crucial to the survival and evolution of the human species (Chuster, 2014, 2018). Utilizing Maturana and Varela's definition of a "living being"[10] (a living being is a cognitive being; hence, it learns from experience), elucidated how this process applies to humans. In their perspective, even a bacterium learns, integrating this learning into its DNA. However, in humans, the learning experience is not encoded in DNA but is allocated to the enigmatic "mind." This underscores the significance of the question Bion consistently posed: What is the mind?

In animals, the learning process stems from an instinctual apprehension of the world. However, in humans, the learning trajectory is fundamentally distinct. Humans embark on a lifelong quest for knowledge and skills from the moment they are born. Bion's pre-conception theory illuminates how human survival is enabled by an evolutionary genetic shift toward *neoteny*—the prolonged retention of juvenile features into adulthood. This retardation in physical maturity has likely permitted the development of distinct human capacities such as advanced emotional communication and enhanced ability to learn from experience, facilitated by improved cognitive processing. This evolutionary trait endows humans with an exceptional ability to adapt and thrive in diverse environments.

The essence of the previous discussion on human beings' ability to learn from experience, in the context of Bion's preconception theory, is as follows: A human infant, born into complete dependence, must undergo a process of learning to survive. This learning, encompassing the full scope of bodily experiences, requires more than mere experimentation; it demands learning from these experiences. To achieve this, one must first master the capacity to think, which extends beyond mere desire. Thinking necessitates enduring the unknown and unexpected, making patience a key foundation for initiating this journey of learning and thinking.

Patience represents the negotiation with our intolerance for the frustration brought about by our thoughts, whether due to their mere nature as thoughts or their inherent tendency to thwart action. It reflects the ability to tolerate the inherent unpredictability of each experience until achieving a state of safety, which manifests as protection, satisfaction, and containment.

In human development, learning from experience emerges when a pre-conception mates with a realization, giving birth to a conception. This is the most primitive step of oedipal theory, in which *Mother pre-conception* mates with *Father realization* to give birth to *baby conception*.

In the earliest stages of human evolution, approximately 6 to 7 million years ago, certain adaptations were essential for enhancing the ability to learn from experience. These changes were crucial for coping with the challenges posed by nomadic lifestyles and an environment inhabited by hostile and formidable predators.

The fundamental theory posits that these adaptations involved a reduction in the impact of innate factors, a concept known as *neoteny*.[11] Consequently, the evolutionary trajectory of pre-human offspring led to their being born increasingly less developed, thereby minimizing the influence of innate predispositions and augmenting the potential for experiential learning.

This foundation for a new level of achievement has become encoded within human DNA, equipping humans with enhanced adaptability to diverse environments and, notably, the ability to develop technologies for predator defense. What was once predominantly innate is now largely confined to physical form and functions. Distinct from other mammals and species, humans learn from experience and record these learnings in the enigmatic construct known as the "mind."

From these rudimentary yet complex conditions emerged the social-historical world; groups and organizations formed with the purpose of safeguarding immature offspring until they reached maturity. However, this immaturity can never be fully eradicated. Our species maintains a level of underdevelopment that Bion refers to as the *embryonic mind*, essential for the plasticity necessary in a thinking being.

The unceasing amplification of group significance has transitioned the human milieu from nature to society. This societal characteristic constitutes another inborn root of the species, suggesting that humans are inherently destined to be both social and mental beings. These attributes proliferate through the experience of culture, whose expansion hinges on the preservation of the value of pre-conception even after their transformation into conceptions and concepts.

The previously mentioned mathematical definition of "realization" involves *the succession of infinite sets with the repetition of signs*. This notion aligns closely with Matte Blanco's theories on the unconscious as comprising infinite sets.[12] The overarching idea is the application of theory of functions to establish links between these infinite sets.[13]

Applying modern concepts of complexity to living organizations enables the conceptualization of a model of the *embryonic mind*, through a blend of fiction and analogy, drawing on theories like the existence of a fourth natural force: the *electroweak* force.[14] The interaction of this force with primordial life forms (amino acid clusters), acting as particles that reveal latent symmetries, enabled these life forms to self-organize and navigate through chaotic circumstances. Within the amniotic fluid of the womb, such forces might have offered novel organizational pathways to the pre-human fetus. Thus, it is plausible that numerous societal influences[15] could signal symmetries for the embryo to emulate.

Employing this model makes it possible to imaginatively conjecture that a significant element could be the rhythms present in the prenatal environment (Chuster, 2014, 2018). These rhythms, representing space-time experiences, serve to open a window (pre-conception) to the world. In other words, prenatal rhythms function as indicators of hidden symmetries, akin to *strange attractors*.[16] However, I believe a more suitable term for this phenomenon might be *radical imagination,* as proposed by Castoriadis (1997).[17]

Radical imagination, as outlined by Chuster (1999, 2002, 2005b, 2014, 2018c), posits that pre-conception possesses an inherent component that shapes the human essence through bodily morphology and an immutable core that evolves into the mind. Notably, its openness, stemming from a degree of immaturity, facilitates a spectrum of developmental outcomes, ranging from creative to perverse, and from productive to destructive. This spectrum extends to the social, fostering social autonomy and to the narcissistic, leading to a loss of freedom and various expressions of tyranny.

This chapter concludes with selected quotations from Bion on the subject:

Embryologists can talk about 'optic pits' and 'auditory pits.' Is it possible for us, as psychoanalysts, to think that it can be traces in the human being, which would suggest the survival, in the human mind, similar to those in the human body, of indications, in the optic field, that in a certain period there were optical pits, or in the hearing field, that in a certain moment there were auditory pits? Is there any part of the human mind that still has signs of an "embryonic" intuition, be it visual or auditory? Is there any connection between the thought and the emotional life post-natal... should we think that the fetus thinks, or feels, or sees, or hears? If there is like this, how primitive can these thoughts, feelings, or ideas be?[18]

The first and foremost of these imaginative conjectures is that adrenal glands do not think, but the structures that surround them develop in the physical prediction to fulfill the functions that we know as thinking and feeling. The embryo or its optic, auditory, and adrenal pits do not see, hear, fight nor run away, but the body develops in the prediction of having to provide the apparatus that will perform the functions of thinking, seeing, hearing, running away, and so on.[19]

Notes

1 W.R. Bion, "Introduction," *Transformations*, 1965, Karnac Books.
2 W.R. Bion, *Transformations*, 1965, Karnac Books, p. 12.
3 W.R. Bion, *Learning from Experience*, 1962b, Karnac Books, pp. 69–70.
4 A joke typically starts our meetings of the Bion Study Group, *Free Bion!* One of the members, Karen Willette, created a coffee cup emblazoned with this phrase and gifted it to each group member: James and Shirley Gooch, Kirby Ogden, Thomas Helscher, Marianne Robinson, Robin Goldberg, Afsaneh Alisobhani, Arnoldo Chuster, and Glenda Corstorphine.
5 Another approach to comprehending the evolution of conceptions into concepts is provided by the theory of internal objects. This theory posits that an internal object results from a multifaceted process involving not just Realization, but also various functions of the individual's mind. However, the Theory of Thinking extends beyond the scope of internal objects theory, holding a different epistemological status. Therefore, I opt to retain the terminology of conceptions and concepts to fully capture the complexity we aim to elucidate throughout this book.

6 Note that the traditional concept of analytical treatment, rooted in the medical model, has undergone a complete transformation. Psychoanalysis can be conceptualized as a human capacity that the analytical process aids in developing. This capacity cannot be imparted to someone as though it were a medication. Following Bion, the role of analysts has evolved into a more modest one. Our primary function is to facilitate the development of this capacity, the psychoanalytic function of the personality, in our analysands.

7 Editor's note, "*Constant Conjunction*" is employed in philosophy to denote a concept closely related to causality and induction, often serving as a near synonym. Its application frequently challenges the adage "correlation does not imply causality." This term is closely associated with Hume due to his extensive exploration of the limits of empiricism in his discussions on causality and inference.

8 A. Chuster, *A Lonesome Road: Essays on the Complexity of W.R. Bion's Work*, 2014, Trio Studio, Grafica Digital, Chapter 9, "The Myth of Satan," p. 175.

9 W. Stegmaier, *Friedrich Nietzsche zur Einführung*, 2nd ed., 2013, Hamburg, Junius.

10 H. Maturana and F. Varela, *Autopoiesis and Cognition: The Realization of Living*, 1991, Springer Science & Business Media.

11 David B. Wake, "What Salamanders Have Taught Us About Evolution." *Annual Review of Ecology, Evolution, and Systematics*, 40, December, 2009, pp. 333–352. DOI:0.1146/annurev.ecolsys.39.110707.173552.

12 I. Matte Blanco, *The Unconscious as Infinite Sets: An Essay in Bi-logic*, 1980, Karnac Books.

13 Editor's note, this idea will be explored in more detail in Chapter 10.

14 D. J. Griffiths, *Introduction to Elementary Particles*, 1987, John Wiley & Sons Inc.; W. Greiner and B. Müller, *Gauge Theory of Weak Interactions*, 2000, Springer; and G. L. Kane, *Modern Elementary Particle Physics*, 1987, Perseus Books.

15 Editor's note, in previous works, the author has elucidated the external influences on fetal development, highlighting how the mother's daily routines and her interactions with family and society at large create a multifaceted environment. This complex milieu, both intra-uterine and extra-uterine, significantly impacts the fetus's progression into infancy.

16 An attractor is a set of numerical values toward which a system tends to evolve. When an attractor possesses a fractal structure and is dependent on its to initial conditions, it is termed "strange and chaotic." The Lorenz system serves as a key example of this concept. The notion of a strange attractor illustrates that trajectories converging towards this attractor are highly sensitive to their starting point. Lorenz's research into chaotic phenomena culminated in the development of a concept of singularity within such events, underscoring the significant impact of minor variations in systems where predictability becomes impossible due to turbulence.

17 Editor's note, Cornelius Castoriadis, a Greek-French philosopher, economist, social critic, and psychoanalyst, was the author of *The Imaginary Institution of Society*. His oeuvre can be understood broadly as a reflection on the concept of creativity, autonomy and social institutions.

18 W.R. Bion, *The Grid and Caesura*, 1975, Imago, Rio de Janeiro.

19 W.R. Bion, *Clinical Seminars and Four Papers*, 1990, Routledge.

Chapter 10

Realization

The Complex Transformations of Pre-conception to Conception

This chapter delves into the complex link between mathematical concepts and psychoanalysis, fostering a dialogue between *rational* and *imaginative conjectures* to construct a model of Realization through the vertex of complexity. This dialogue intends to provide a pragmatic example of Bion's theory of thinking, leading to the elucidation of concepts encapsulated within the term "transformations."

> The changes I have had to make throughout this book from analogy to more precise formulation, and from more precise formulation again, illustrate some of the difficulties with which I am attempting to deal. All these changes are examples of transformation.[1]

The preceding chapter succinctly articulated the mathematical definition of Realization[2] as a *succession of infinite sets with a repetition of signs*. These "signs" are *proto-symbols* in the embryonic mind, undergoing transformations until they become symbols in the post-natal mind by means of reverie/alpha function.

Symbols are either autonomous or heteronymous, as delineated by Meltzer (1996). *Heteronymous* symbols, integral to Culture, represent tools and concepts universally shared among individuals. In contrast, *autonomous* symbols are personal creations, emerging from psychic processes that characterize individual conceptions and subjectivity.

I consider the process of realization according to the imaginative conjectures as proposed by Bion's later works, envisaging it as a two-staged movement separated by a caesura.[3] This concept underscores the continuity between the inaccessible pre-natal, embryonic mind—ruled by chance, indetermination and random potentiality—and the post-natal mind, a realm of constant experimentations ruled by choices. Together, these stages delineate the universe of complexity.

The infinite sets[4] are very specific in each stage of Realization. Whether pre-natal (rhythms) or post-natal (symbols), each stage harbors an inaccessible and enigmatic origin, emblematic of inherent complexity.

Bion employed John Milton's aesthetic phrase *"the void and formless infinite"* to represent "O," the core of all transformations hitherto discussed. "O," akin to

DOI: 10.4324/9781003474128-11

an "original pre-conception" (Chuster, 1997a), operates within the embryonic mind. In a state of expectation, it functions as a psychic frame to a "window-to-the-world." This preview of the world anticipates receiving a "picture of the world" through post-natal experiences (Chuster, 2014, 2018a, 2018b).

These time-space frames originate from intra-uterine rhythmic patterns: the symphony of the baby's and mother's heartbeats, the rhythm of the bladder, and intestinal peristalsis, are all subtly influenced by the mother's daily activities. The assortment of tones, timbres, and rhythmic forms functions akin to an orchestra rehearsing for the inaugural ceremony of birth, guided by the routines and vicissitudes of the expectant mother's life. Moreover, a manifested plethora of incidents, coincidences, and conflicts in syncopated, dissonant beats. These rhythms and backbeats, particularly in the maternal link with herself and the fetus, are experiential imprints. This process undoubtedly illustrates how Culture permeates the unborn child within the womb, a realm far from insulated from these multifaceted experiences.

In the embryonic phase of Realization, we can postulate that highly sensorial *infinite sets* such as touch, smell,[5] hearing,[6] and movement operate as formative elements within the formless space of the womb. Their intensity and diverse combinations contribute to shaping the pre-natal frames that form pre-conception in its most primitive form.

However, limiting the discussion to only these four sensory operators does not adequately capture the model's complexity. Daily life presents immense variability, leading to an extensive array of possible operational combinations. According to the Uncertainty principle, even this basic four-to-four ratio does not circumvent the epistemological necessity. In other words, every theory one creates must be open and undeniably incomplete. Beyond these four sets lies an *empty* set, related to the μ factor of the psychoanalytic object, representing the complexity of this object. Consequently, one must contend with a minimum range of combinations, extending from five to infinity.

The outcome of these *infinite set*[7] combinations traverse the birth's caesura and recombine with new sets of high sensory intensity. Freud's model of libido development—oral, anal, and phallic stages—represents experiences shaping our worldview, further detailed in Karl Abraham's theory. While these developmental theories provide a reference frame, Bion's theory, focusing on observation or perception, necessitates a different theoretical approach.

The same epistemological features of an open system are applicable to the pre-natal stage, therefore, an empty set (staying open to an everlasting mystery) should be included as a theoretical guide to observations of the post-natal phase of Realization, thus allowing for combinations ranging from a minimum of five sensorial sets to an infinite array of experiences. This underscores the undeniable singularity and complexity of human experience.

The "spectrum model reverie/alpha function" operates from birth in the caesura between minds, endeavoring to "digest" the interaction of set combinations traversing from one realm to another. The μ factor (complexity) introduces indeterminacy into our observational perspectives, allowing for infinite combinations and leading Bion to propose substituting the dynamics between *conscious ↔ unconscious* with *infinite ↔ finite*.

An additional epistemological consideration is the theoretical status of pre-conception movement in the embryonic mind. Since movements in the prenatal mind cannot be classified as projective identification (lacking an object), a different terminology is suggested. Drawing on Cornelius Castoriadis' ideas, I (Chuster 1999, 2002, 2014, 2018) proposed the term *"radical imagination"* for prenatal movements, reserving "projective identification" for post-birth interactions involving an object.

Before birth, in the absence of objects, there is only the formation of a space-time frame, an empty frame, which develops to receive and engage with post-natal images and experiences. Premature object formation in this phase can lead to a primitive, blind, and rigid picture, potentially resulting in conditions like autism or schizophrenia, characterized by unyielding patterns and a disoriented or non-existent worldview.

Acknowledging the concept of *no-object* (no-thing) and the lifelong presence of the embryonic mind within us necessitates a reevaluation of the theoretical framework for the reception of experiences for the analytical practice. I (Chuster, 2014, 2018) propose moving beyond Freud's developmental libido theory to adopt two general levels of experience: an *aesthetic level* linked to emotional life and initial sensorial (including now visual) experiences, and an *ethical level*, where these experiences acquire values based on choices. These levels combine to form *conceptions*, inherently containing aesthetic and ethical components, a status maintained even as they evolve into concepts. Group experiences introduce common sense and moral dimensions, often leading to conflicts in life values.

In light of these conflicts, the question of what constitutes ethical values becomes pertinent. This fundamental query might address different ethics, such as survival ethics, life ethics, or business ethics, among others, and is central to understanding patient's experiences.

An important feature of psychoanalytic ethics is not to doubt the accuracy, sincerity, or the authenticity of a patient's observations, whether they involve, for instance, perceptions of external hostility or internalized conspiracies, but rather the interpretation and understanding of these experiences within their unique psychological framework. For instance, when a patient says that the neighbor's dog is barking because of him; or asserts that he hears conspiring voices coming from the television, or believes that a hacker has downloaded these voices into his head, or feels that the radio is making veiled accusations about homosexuality, should we say he is not right or these beliefs are a distortion produced by conflicts?

Surely, the patient knows more about his experiences than the analyst does. Our task is to perceive beyond the immediate, to listen beyond the words, and to keep our imagination open to the echoes of primitive mental states. This pursuit presents years of intricate work, necessitating what Bion called *"the act of faith"* (1970): a commitment to seeking truth.

It is worth discussing in this part of the chapter the link between pre-natal radical imagination and post-natal imagination (driven by projective identification), leading up to subjectivity and social imagination (conceptions and concepts).

In early post-natal life, the mother's reverie ruptures the infant's closed psychic world. That is, the mother's mind, through her reverie, initiates the baby's *socialization*. This process is supported not only by the mother's mind but also by the combined mental influence of both parents. Beyond the mind of the sexually united parents lies the influence of the family and, further still, the broader society, which creates conditions conducive to the development of creative minds to meet various needs of the babies. In complexity theory, this is termed "auto-poietic looping," a never-ending cycle that traverses beyond all known facts.

The maternal function (reverie), from the point of view of human evolution, represents a culmination of 6 to 4 million years of *hominization* process, and it remains open to further evolution. This statement does not invalidate the mother's unconscious and unique singularity that influence the child. However, the unconscious itself is shaped by the mother's socialization process, integral to her ability to nurture and teach the child to think and speak. However, over millions of years, these abilities have evolved, varying infinitely from individual to individual.

In analytic practice, the starting point of observation involves a specific mental state devoid of memory and desire (or negative capability), linking blind intuitions with empty concepts. The analyst's mind strives to link imaginative conjectures with rational ones, fostering progressive inquiries toward achieving interpretative language. Initial intuitions apprehend the rhythms conveyed by the analysand, while concepts are drawn from selected theories to contain these most primitive perceptions of the transient material.

Freud recognized, after a quarter-century, that for psychoanalytic practice, knowledge in literature, ethnology, history, philosophy, and archaeology was more crucial than medicine. This assertion, supported in *"The Question of Lay Analysis"* (1926)[8], implies that a psychoanalyst must be proficient in these fields to comprehend language phenomena (meanings). Bion (1970) regarded Freud's work as an embodiment of the *"Language of Achievement"*: a language that is both a *prelude to action* and a *type of action itself*. It serves as a prelude, facilitating preparation for future situations. Simultaneously, it is an action—in the here and now of the analytic session—engaging with phenomena that emerge and become evident through the process of thinking. This duality perpetuates a complex circularity between action and prelude.

Complexity in Bion's *Theory of Thinking* (1962a) introduced an unusual epistemological notion, which can be referred to as the *implicate order*. Derived from Latin, this term implies to "involve." Divergent with the explicative order (which is more prevalent in traditional psychoanalytic culture), the implicate order views the analytical process as a generator of thinking aimed not just at acquiring knowledge, but also at transformative knowledge. This encompasses knowledge of the self, fostering personal transformation, *"becoming one self,"* with aspects that often challenge verbal expression.

In Bion (1965), this concept is illustrated as "*transformation in O*," where the emotional experience of transformation exemplifies the complexity of the implicate order.

The combination of psychic sets leads to experiences that evolve from conceptions to the formation of a concept, a representation of a worldview facilitating social links many times by common sense. For instance, the dimensions of an isolated concept, like "inside" and "outside," might clearly manifest in dreams, reflecting conflicts between ethical and moralistic values or the impact of group morality on natural human ethics. An implicate order creates circularity between inside and outside by means of a caesura.

A picture of the world,[9] shaped by conceptions and concepts, represents an expansion of thoughts, feelings, and ideas, including those arising from failures, delusions, beliefs, false conceptions, and lies. For instance, a worldview dominated by visual sets may offer an emotional and aesthetic perspective on reality. Yet, this view could adopt an "aesthetic of evil" if, in its realization, it competes with tactile sets. Similarly, a worldview prioritizing rationality and control could devolve into a perverse view of reality if it competes with the kinetic sets (sense of movement).

The challenge lies in observing symmetries like rationality and perversion, generosity and complacency, joy and euphoria, or helplessness and omnipotence, which will be explored in future discussions.

These are merely a few of the infinite combinations produced by Realization. Each analyst must establish a singular spectrum for capturing these possibilities, always applying the *Principle of Uncertainty*[10] to their observations.

Notes

1 W.R. Bion, *Transformations*, 1965, Karnac Books, p. 119.
2 T. Dreyfus, *Advanced Mathematical Thinking Processes*, 2016, Mathematics Education Library, Springer.
3 "Let us take a flight into fantasy, a species of the childhood of our thought. I can imagine a situation in which the fetus, ready to be born, could be aware of extremely unpleasant oscillations in the amniotic fluid before moving to the gaseous medium – in other words, the birth. I can imagine that there is some disturbance happening, for example, a disagreement between the parents. I can keep imagining very loud noises coming from the father and the motheror noises made by the mother's digestive system. Imagine that the fetus is also aware of the pressures from something that one day will become a character or a personality aware of elements such as fear, hate, primitive emotions. Then, I think that the fetus could, in an omnipotent way, transform these disturbing feelings into hostility, proto-ideas, proto-feelings, and in a very precocious stage, split them up, destroy them, and try to excrete them. I suppose, then, when the baby is subjected to the birth trauma and to the immediate trauma of having to adjust to the gaseous medium (one way of doing that is bringing with him/her the aqueous medium, in order to preserve this capacity of secreting mucus and, hence, continuing to smell, since some internal fluids allow some olfactory centers to keep working). I can imagine that the fetus is so precocious, so premature, that he/she tries to get rid of his/her personality." W.R. Bion, 1976.
4 Infinite set theory encompasses proofs and definitions central to understanding its complexity. Key concepts include defining "elements" or components of a set, distinguishing

unique elements within a set, and establishing proofs of infinity. The theory elaborates on various types of infinity, such as countable and uncountable sets. When contrasting infinite with finite sets, topics such as ordered sets, cardinality, equivalency, coordinate planes, universal sets, mapping, subsets, continuity, and transcendence are pivotal. Cantor's foundational ideas in set theory were notably influenced by trigonometry and the concept of irrational numbers.

5 "The sense of smell is a receptor that works afar in aqueous fluid. Sharks and groupers provide a model of this receptor that works afar, but the human being has to bring this intracellular fluid after birth to a world where the medium is not aqueous but gaseous. Instead of being an advantage, the aqueous fluid may become inadequate, the person complains of what medical doctors call rhinitis, which causes breathing difficulties."

embryonic / olfactory $\Big\langle$———————— Realization —————–$\Big\rangle$ post – natal / rhinitis

6 "The embryologists affirm that the optic and auditory pits appear in the third somite. I do not want to suggest that, due to this fact, the fetus would be able to see or to hear around this age. It would be more plausible if he/she were a fetus ready to be born. However, which would be an epoch when is reasonable to suppose that the eyes and ears started to work? I had no difficulty to suppose that there are pressure oscillations in the amniotic fluid – after all the fluid can transmit waves, of variable lengths, which impact any receptor organ that is present."

7 In *The Unconscious as Infinite Sets*, Matte Blanco identifies two distinct modes of relational logic: *Symmetric*, which he aligns with symmetrical logic, and *Asymmetric*, corresponding to bivalent logic. Conscious thought predominantly operates within the realm of bivalent logic, where relationships are irreversible and propositions are strictly true or false—hence asymmetrical. This logic underpins the clear demarcation between object and subject, and the differentiation of individuals through unique relationships and reality testing. For example, in bivalent logic, if "X is larger than Y," the converse cannot be true.

Conversely, symmetric logic typifies the unrepressed unconscious, challenging conscious cognition with its complexity. In this mode, elements are interchangeable and capable of being reversed to their symmetric opposite, nullifying individual identities and perceiving entities as members of classes or classes of classes. Within symmetric logic, a paradox emerges, such as "Y is simultaneously larger and smaller than X." However, in the repressed unconscious, elements retain vestiges of asymmetry from their previous conscious processing. Matte Blanco introduces the concept of *bi-logic*, the coexistence of symmetric and asymmetric logics in all psychic phenomena. The prevalence of symmetry over asymmetry in this blend dictates the unconscious degree of the phenomenon.

Furthermore, Matte Blanco expands upon Klein's insight, equating the sentiment "I am angry with X" with "Someone is angry with me." He acknowledges Klein as one of the most innovative and original thinkers inspired by Freud, especially for her renowned concept of projective identification. For Matte Blanco, the essence of unconsciousness is symmetry, characterized by a propensity for "sameness" and a concurrent aversion to difference.

8 In late spring of 1926, Theodor Reik, a prominent non-medical member of the Vienna Psychoanalytic Society, was charged with a breach of an old Austrian law against quackery—a law which made it illegal for non-physicians to treat patients. Freud at once intervened and penned "*The Question of Lay Analysis*" in his support. This work, structured as an informal dialogue with an "impartial interlocutor"—likely Julius Tandler, a Viennese city councilor for welfare with whom Freud had discussed Reik's situation—addressed the longstanding issue of "lay" analysis within Freud's circle. This debate centered on whether psychoanalysis should be restricted to physicians. Freud and some of his followers, valuing thorough analytical training over medical qualifications, diverged from others, notably Abraham A. Brill and American counterparts, who

viewed analysis strictly as a medical discipline and advocated barring non-physicians from its practice.

Ernest Jones, recognizing the significance of this divide, conducted an extensive survey within the analytic community. This culminated in 28 presentations at the Innsbruck International Congress in September 1927, though no consensus emerged. Freud, persisting in his stance, penned a "Postscript" for the event, reiterating his belief in the legitimacy of non-physicians practicing psychoanalysis. S. Freud, SE, Vol. XX, pp. 179–258.

9 Roger Money-Kyrle, *Man's Picture of The World and Three Papers*, edited by Meg Harris Williams, 2015, Karnac Books.

10 Joseph B. Kadane, *Principles of Uncertainty*, 2011, Carnegie Mellon University, Pittsburgh, Chapman and Hall/CRC.

Chapter 11

The Ethical-Aesthetical Principle of Uncertainty

Cultivating New Spaces for Thinking

Applying the Principle of Uncertainty in psychoanalytic observation, inherently intertwined with the Theory of Complexity, necessitates an epistemological understanding of mathematical structures like *Hilbert Space*.[1] This is crucial for managing endless non-linear successions and selecting from multiple operators within this space.

> Heisenberg's Uncertainty principle is an important stage in the journey; it is deplorable that any section of humankind should be certain. If there is anything which is certain it is that certainty is wrong.[2]

The epistemology of a Hilbert space presents a foundational proposition, which can be used in psychoanalysis: the construction of a field that acknowledges its own limits and possibilities. This involves expanding psychoanalytic proposals while concurrently delineating their scope. This concept is a cornerstone in Bion's theory of thinking (1962a), advocating for a new approach to psychoanalysis. It challenges the notion of accommodating observations and concepts within a traditional, definitive space, as no theory or concept is final.

Psychoanalysis, inherently, cannot be a traditional, closed system. It must perpetually open and evolve through practical experience. The application of the principle of complexity to psychoanalysis consistently reinforces this dynamic. This approach often requires enduring and accepting, for a necessary duration, insuperable contradictions, disquieting complexities, inextricable clutter, ambiguity, and, most critically, the inherent uncertainty in any form.

Freud consistently acknowledged the transient nature of his theoretical concepts and was cautious about constructing a systematic, *a priori* analytical experience. In developing analytical concepts, he often highlighted their metaphorical nature. For instance, he regarded the concept of drives as fictional and never asserted the Ego as a reality. He also emphasized the conventional design of the psychic apparatus and steered clear of adapting psychoanalysis to transient trends and fashions. Understanding Freud's need to tailor his formulations to diverse audiences and purposes is key to grasping the complexity embedded in the various layers of his thought.

DOI: 10.4324/9781003474128-12

When Bion (1965) conceptualized the mind using points, lines, curves, and hyperboles, he aligned his thinking with the principles of Hilbert space. This space, an extension of Euclidean space, is not confined to a finite number of dimensions and angles. It is a vector space endowed with an inner product, allowing for variations in distance and angles. In psychoanalytic terms, it is an analogy with the theory of projective identification (representing distance) and the theory of multiple vertices (representing angles).

This approach in psychoanalysis makes it possible to ascertain, from an alternative vertex, the necessity of engaging with transformations. This implies that working with functions (encompassing concepts such as reverie, alpha function, reversal of alpha function, intuitive function, the psychoanalytic function of the personality, elements of psychoanalysis, the Grid, the caesura) necessitates a mental representation of a vector space inherently involving transformations. Consequently, studying transformations in non-linear spaces becomes essential for functional analysis. This forms a circular argument: functions necessitate transformations, which require non-linear space, which again calls for functions and transformations.

Mathematically, operating in a non-linear pathway is feasible through the premise of the *Fourier transform*,[3] which concerns the study of differential and integral equations. The term "functional," in this context, refers to the study of variations, implying the uncertainty and transience of observations. In psychoanalysis, by analogy, this is represented as:

$$T = f\left(\alpha\right). \int i\,/\,v. \left(a \leftrightarrow p\right) = K \rightarrow O$$

This formula conveys that analytic transformation (T) is a product of the alpha function (fα) working to integrate the variables (v) and invariants (i) within the analyst/patient link (a ↔ p), potentially leading to an analytic transformation (K → O). The terms of the equation are inseparable, emphasizing the necessity of integration ($\int$).

The purpose of this mode of thought, though it may seem unconventional to many psychoanalysts, is to underscore the complexity of mental operations within the analytical field. The mathematical expression serves as both a dreamlike feature and imaginative tool, facilitating a psychoanalytic construction.

At the start of *Transformations* (1965), Bion introduces this complexity by drawing a parallel to the images produced by a painter. He likens the psychoanalyst to a painter before their canvas, suggesting a convergence of art, mathematics, and psychoanalysis in a profound contemplation of the observational model.

Suppose a painter sees a path through a field sown with puppies and paints it: at one end of the chain of events is the field of poppies, at the other a canvas with pigment disposed on its surface.[4]

Note that one of the fundamental elements of this chain of events is the scrutiny of the painter (Figure 11.1).

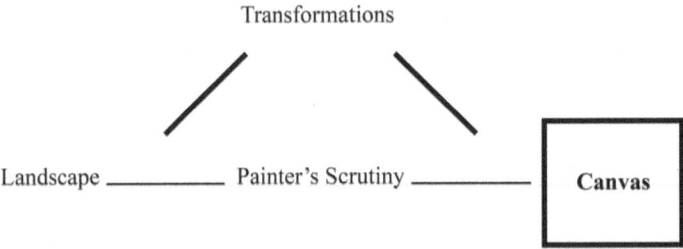

Figure 11.1 Elements in Transformation.

The painting, despite the singular transformations of the painter's perspective, still represents the poppy field. The recognition of the poppy field hinges on certain unaltered elements during the transformation: the *invariants*. The painter, based on his singular perspective, selects these invariants.

In this artistic process, the invariants only represent one crucial element. During interpretation, the painter's choices inevitably omit certain aspects, and these omissions are often a reflection of the artist's unique style and personal perspective. What the painter perceives and fails to perceive is revealed on the canvas. Initially, observers see what their eyes can find on the painting. A dialogue with the painter will be required to uncover other elements beyond this common visual perception. However, in its footsteps, this dialogue reveals an infinite reality that plunges into the unknown.

In a scenario akin to that of an artist, the psychoanalyst engages with a patient who shares a series of events related to their psychic pain. Employing the methodological approach of analytic work, the analyst listens attentively, endeavoring to transform these observations into an interpretive language. At one end of this spectrum is the patient's narrative, and at the other, the analyst's interpretation. Central to this process is the analyst's "look"—a selective perception of invariants in the patient's account, which are then reformed into an interpretation. There is an expectation that the patient recognizes himself in the interpretation. However, an element of uncertainty invariably arises: something remains unaddressed, something is always left out. This omission, or the presence of an absence, alters the dynamic of the observation.

The critical question here is whether this omission stems from the inherent uncertainty of observation or if it represents something the analyst could not confront. This distinction is pivotal. Is it a matter of a blind spot, or an inherent incompleteness in the observational process? Does it reflect a complexity or (counter-trans)-ference?[5] Each possibility carries significant implications for the analytical process and outcome.

Let us consider some clinical material. A patient describes his life as "*a fraud*" or "*a joke*," appearing as if acting out on a stage or circus arena. He conveys this with a bitter, derogatory, and somewhat ironic tone. He seems almost convinced, yet a flicker of uncertainty appears, justifying another attempt when the analyst inquires why he is considering analysis after having had several failed analytic experiences.

During the last one, he convinced his analyst of the necessity for psychiatric medication. This intervention was initially effective, highlighting the limitations of what he referred to as his "ego resources." However, its efficacy was short-lived, indicating he imposed conditions on his treatment, seeking only what he desired to hear.

His pervasive pessimism could be visually conceptualized and interpreted as akin to a drug produced by his mind, possibly leading to a state of melancholia. No medication is potent enough to fight the shadow of a lost object casting over his soul.

The first notable aspect is the patient's denial of a symmetrical perception of himself as both actor and spectator of his life; he excludes himself from scenarios where he is, in fact, the creator. However, it is important to acknowledge that he might perceive his new analysis yet another "comedy." What evidence exists to suggest this new analysis would deviate from the pattern of failures?

When the analyst highlights the potential recurrence of this "comedy," the patient shares the pain associated with his role as a teacher. The act of engaging with his students, akin to stepping onto a stage, is a source of discomfort. He feels torn between being an actor and a spectator.

The analyst explores his tendency for generalization, which transforms his audience into harsh critics, mirroring his own critical nature. Despite this, he perceives himself as fragile and insecure, burdened by feelings of being a "*fraud.*" Gradually, these painful feelings evolve into "*panic,*" a profound fear of interaction and vulnerability, stemming from a deep-seated sense of isolation with seemingly no escape. This loneliness can only have meanings in a symmetry with a dependence on others. However, could this loneliness be a result of feeling excluded as a by-product of a certain perspective on life?

His professional obligation to write papers is overshadowed by his belief in their lack of originality. He perceives himself as a mere imitator with no purpose. Yet, even if the ideas are not entirely his, does he not impart a personal interpretation to them? This raises questions about authorship: Who is truly excluded from the stage—the author, the actor, or the spectator? How do these three roles interact and diverge? What is the nature of their disconnection, and how can what has been fragmented be reintegrated?

It seems that the patient's fear is rooted in the potential exposure of the painful feelings of dependency and loneliness. His sense of being a "fraud" simultaneously reveals and conceals these truths. In his perspective, only something wholly truthful can be considered complete. Since everything is incomplete, he concludes that everything is fraudulent.

Let us explore the vertex of theater analogy further. What do actors do when they portray a character? They give voice to the words of the absent author and bring their text to life. They create a semblance of reality, briefly convincing the audience of its truth. However, what is this truth? Bion (1977a) remarked, "We probably cannot wait for an answer, because we have not the time."

The question might be: where should we look for truth? Not the philosophical truth, but truth about being a human, embodying respect for life, as the ultimate truth.

Alternatively, acknowledging the improbability of discovering absolute truth, what value does such a pursuit hold? Both psychoanalysts and theater practitioners grapple with this dilemma. They engage with an elusive yet central element, akin to an absence that is uncovered through interpretation. This represents a creative process, a work in progress in pursuit of truth, fostering development. Conversely, evading this quest may lead to falsehoods and cruelty, which are transformations that involve both the creation and the destruction of forms.

Refining the question: what endows a theater scene with the power to rouse someone from a dream, prevalent in both wakefulness and sleep? Conversely, how does one awaken from a dream are unaware of dreaming?

Could psychoanalysis fulfill a similar function? Is it possible to improve someone's dreaming while simultaneously helping them awaken from their nightmares or distressing dreams?

If the patient views themselves solely as an observer of their own life, as if it were unfolding on a stage—a notion, referring to a sense of helplessness—it suggests the existence of symmetries to be revealed. For instance, there is a symmetry between blind intuition and empty concept, actor and spectator, or container and contained. In each case, an invariant is present—the excluded object. Such an object has a specific perspective one might choose to observe. This suggests a sequence: function, transformation, invariants, and complexity.

There are six distinct perspectives to consider, each corresponding to the transformations Bion (1965) described. They also signify varying levels of discord between container and contained, creating an empty space filled with specific effects:

a *Rigid Motion Transformations*: encompassing mistakes and misunderstandings.
b *Projective Transformation*: encompassing mistakes and misunderstandings + falsehoods.
c *Transformation in Hallucinosis*: involving mistakes and misunderstandings + falsehoods + lies.
d *Transformation in K*: this occurs when there is relative harmony in the container/contained relationship.
e *Analytical transformation*, K→O: this happens if the analyst is able to transform K into psychoanalysis.
f *Transformation in O*: this may occur if the patient is able to utilize the analytic transformation.

A detailed examination of transformations in hallucinosis takes into account the container/contained configuration, where decisions hinge on moralistic criteria for inclusion and exclusion. In other words, the core characteristic of these transformations becomes apparent when a patient excludes something, guided by a moralistic viewpoint.

The logic of a moralistic perspective—characterized by dichotomies such as right/wrong, top/bottom, superior/inferior—binds the patient to a harsh judgment of human relationships. Occasionally, this perspective leaves the patient without a comprehensive understanding of what it means to be human.

A patient, from a very young age, set his life's ambition to become an "intellectual," unknowingly driven by a fear of physical experiences, including sexual encounters. This choice entrapped him within a restrictive personal code, initiating a prolonged and expansive cycle of transformation in hallucinosis.

Describing this transformation to the patient involves explaining how he selectively excludes and criticizes anything that does not align with his self-imposed "intellectual code." This means addressing his beliefs that an intellectual should avoid certain behaviors, like attending a gym, dressing fashionably, or engaging with specific types of literature and everyday activities. It is important to highlight how the restrictions he places on himself are expressions of his broader difficulty in processing and integrating experiences—a manifestation of what might be seen as an impaired alpha function.

By dismissing the body's reality, the patient justified engaging in harmful behaviors: substance abuse, excessive alcohol consumption, sleep deprivation, unhealthy eating, loveless relationships, and promiscuous sexual activity, resulting in a life plagued by toxic interactions. Eventually, his body succumbed to the strain, manifesting signs of failure and illness, which challenged his sense of omnipotence.

The false premise (usually not perceived as creating a logic) drives the patient to revere the social code (forming moralistic upper and lower values). However, precisely through this reverence, we can find why he feels excluded. That is when he follows the code to disqualify others and consequently feels that the others will do the same.

The unrecognized, underlying false premise compels the patient to adhere strictly to a reverence for hierarchy, which is subsequently employed to judge others, establishing his criteria for exclusion. This process, in turn, precipitates a fear of reciprocal judgment in a similar vein.

His split perspective enables him to criticize everything deemed superficial, adopting a scornful view toward all that lacks essence. Yet, this perspective overlooks the inherent symmetry between the superficial and the essence, failing to recognize that an essence devoid of appearance is as false as an appearance lacking essence (Bion, 1979). This critical, envious gaze, which could be termed an "evil eye," characterizes transformations in hallucinosis.

The patient exhibits levels of split between his narrative and the truth, both originating from the same point, "O." A caesura separates his story from the truth, introducing a triad: the spectator, the story, and the truth. The links among these elements are subject to varying degrees of severance, contingent on the nature of the transformation influencing them.

Additionally, interpreting the patient's experience through a mythical lens opens up more possibilities. The mythical lens serves as an example of employing Bion's Row C elements.

A *myth* describes passions, invariably including perspectives on the world and its trajectory, as well as humanity and its fate. Myths constitute one of the three domains of application for the psychoanalytic object: myths, senses, and passions.

Every myth represents an attempt to articulate an encounter with "O" through a narrative. Freud utilized the Oedipus myth to unveil psychoanalysis, thereby establishing a precedent for interpreting other myths in different narratives and with distinct characters, all aiming to elucidate the same subject: the human mind.

The Prometheus myth aptly mirrors the patient's predicament: chained to the rock of his moral code, his liver devoured by a divine emissary, a vulture symbolizing his bitterness and overwhelming pessimism, born from his inability to reconcile the divisions wrought in the early tragedy of his life—the tragedy rooted in the failure of the alpha function.

The gods, from whom he stole the flame of knowledge, have exiled the narrative. Their tale can no longer claim authenticity. What persists is merely the absence of evidence to affirm their existence—the absence of the gods' corporeal form. Dionysus, in particular, remains fragmented, symbolizing the absence of the real body. This constitutes his sensation of being an impostor. In other words, incompleteness is not accepted by his omnipotence, therefore, he considers himself a fraud.

The patient left his childhood under severe emotional strain, positioned as a spectator to a past cluttered with buried objects, harboring ongoing, unresolved grief. His endeavors to embody the intellectual, to present well to others, to appear competent, and to maintain a potent image, were merely survival strategies. Yet, these efforts led to a self-imposed alienation, distancing him from his own truth. Consequently, he had not a genuine experience of life. While his crafted story unfolded, the truth lagged behind.

He recounted a dream where he found himself flying over a burial ground. In this dream, he observed a dark, foul-smelling liquid seeping onto the pathways from the graves. Unexpectedly, his capacity to fly diminished, leading him to plummet at the intersection of two streets just beyond the cemetery. He awoke alarmed and unsettled, tormented by the lingering sense of a nightmare's grip.

The analyst highlighted the relevance of the cemetery's name, John the Baptist, in the patient's dream—a biblical character betrayed by Salome, a woman. The patient recently experienced impotence with a woman and feared public shaming on social networks by her. This impotence, a recurring theme (invariant) in his life, mirrors his fear of job loss due to fraud allegations, reflecting his struggles with feelings of omnipotence.

I also called his attention to another detail of the dream in which he fell at a crossroads where there was a street with the same name as the analyst. I tried to show him that he had a choice between falling into his already known depression (his graveyard), which leads to helplessness and persecution or falling into an analysis in which we did not know the outcome. However, we would have some outcome, at least, as another option.

The analyst drew the patient's attention to a detail in his dream where he plummeted at a crossroads, near a street sharing the analyst's name. This was highlighted as a choice between falling into his familiar pattern of depression and feelings of persecution, symbolized by the graveyard, or venturing into the unknown territory of analysis. The latter path did not guarantee a specific outcome, yet it promised the possibility of a different resolution beyond his accustomed despair and vulnerability.

This chapter endeavored to illuminate the psychoanalytic journey as one of perpetual transformation, where the acceptance of uncertainty not only challenges but also enriches our understanding of the self and the other. Through the interplay of functions, transformations, and the quest for truth amidst the complexities of human emotions and relationships, psychoanalysis emerges as a dynamic field ever in flux, embodying the very essence of human exploration and the endless pursuit of understanding. This conceptual framework, embracing the uncertain and the incomplete, propels psychoanalysis into new realms of thought, offering a richer, more nuanced perspective on the intricate tapestry of the human condition.

Notes

1 Hilbert spaces are a fundamental concept in mathematics and physics, commonly manifesting as infinite-dimensional function spaces. These spaces are crucial in various fields, including partial differential equations, quantum mechanics, Fourier analysis (with its practical applications in signal processing and heat transfer), and ergodic theory, which provides the mathematical foundation for thermodynamics. The term "Hilbert space" was coined by John von Neumann to encapsulate the abstract idea central to these diverse applications. The introduction and success of Hilbert-space methods marked a highly productive period in the field of functional analysis. Beyond the traditional Euclidean spaces, Hilbert spaces encompass a variety of examples. These include spaces of square-integral functions, spaces of sequences, Sobolev spaces, which consist of generalized functions, and Hardy spaces that are made up of holomorphic functions. Each of these spaces illustrates the versatility and wide-ranging utility of Hilbert spaces in mathematical and physical theories.

2 Chris Mawson (ed.), *The Complete Works of W.R. Bion*, Vol. VIII, 2014, Karnac Books, p. 342.

3 The Fourier transform is a mathematical technique that decomposes a time-based function, such as a signal, into its constituent frequencies. This process is analogous to breaking down a musical chord into the individual frequencies or pitches of its notes. The result of is a complex-valued function of frequency. The absolute value of this function indicates the intensity of a particular frequency in the original function, while its complex argument denotes the phase offset of the basic sinusoid at that frequency. The Fourier transform is commonly referred to as the *frequency domain representation* of the original signal.

4 W.R. Bion, *Transformations*, 1965, Karnac Books, p. 1.

5 Bion, W. R. (1977a). Two Papers: *The Grid and Caesura*, ed. J. Salomao. Rio de Janeiro: Imago Editora. (Revised edition London: Karnac, 1989.), p. 41.

Chapter 12

The Spectrum Model (Open Systems)[1] and the Diverse Grids

The foundational premise of this chapter posits that each spectrum model represents an *open system*. Bion's work offers a continuum of such models, notably exemplified by the *psychotic/non-psychotic parts of the personality* spectrum (Bion, 1956). Additional instances include the reverie/alpha function, the *narcissism/social-ism spectrum* of the psychoanalytic object, the open observational Grid model, the memory/desire spectrum, and the subsequent caesura model. This latter model, delineating the pre-natal/post-natal spectrum, serves to elucidate various transitional mental states encountered in the analytical process, including dream/awake, transference/countertransference, and transitive/intransitive humor.

> It sometimes helps to illuminate an analytic problem by speaking of a characteristic as appearing to the patient a ghost of the past. The infant experiences what may be called ghosts of the future. Such locutions are possible to adult investigations for maturity provides terms born of experience together with facility in their manipulation. But the facts of personality, its own and that of others, exist for the infant and present him with problems that he must solve.[2]

The paradigm shifts induced by this model introduce a remarkably intriguing epistemological perspective. It departs from the classic structural model in psychoanalysis that relies on a system of classification leading to a diagnosis—a framework that expands over time to sustain its logical architecture. Contrary to discussing neuroses, perversions, extensive classifications, or structural issues, Bion's approach focuses on delineating a spectrum of psychotic and non-psychotic parts of the personality, eschewing any deterministic logical structures.

This subject has various angles to highlight critical aspects of understanding Bion's psychoanalytic model, beginning with the epistemological perspective.

Philosophers of science pay particular attention to the significance of scientific revolutions, which are initiated by geniuses—individuals whose capabilities and, importantly, imagination compel the scientific community to relinquish old patterns of thought in favor of novel and uncharted concepts. While placing less emphasis on changes in working style, it is recognized that in the realm of scientific

DOI: 10.4324/9781003474128-13

progress, shifts in methodology could be as influential as the innovations introduced by a conventional genius.

Bion embodies both elements highlighted in the discussion on scientific revolutions within the realm of psychoanalysis. His approach has a unique blend of
humorous reverence and pointed critique of the knowledge obtained through psychoanalysis. This approach stems from a perspective he articulates on multiple
occasions: life defies precision and conventionality. According to Bion, human existence is rooted in Thinking, a process that reflects our emotions and necessitates
the ability to integrate these emotions. Furthermore, it demands the adoption of
principles that can translate prudence into action (1979).

The last statement serves as a *caveat*, safeguarding our practice. It acts as a
"guardian angel" for the analyst, forming an ethical barrier that underpins the at-
tentive listening and subsequent interpretations. This is crucial because psychoanalysis ranks among the most intricate and challenging endeavors in the human
domain, melding nuanced and abstract concepts that often defy comprehension,
utilizing a technical complexity that is never fully mastered (Chuster, 2018a).

Bion's unique methodological style has deep roots in his personal life, marked
by diverse, challenging, and complex experiences. He often appeared to view the
world through the lens of a vast children's game, reminiscent of "snakes and ladders," a tasteful extension of his childhood in India. This perspective captures the
dynamic interplay of virtues (ladders) and vices (snakes), influencing our decisions
toward either growth or deterioration—a theme that invariably emerges at some
juncture in psychoanalytic exploration.

I perceive the Grid as akin to a game of decisions and choices, influenced by
personal virtues and vices. It serves both as a reflection of the inquiries posed in
Rudyard Kipling's poem, "*The Elephant's Child*,"[3] and as an illustration of how
Bion's childhood reflections evolved into a refined instrument.

Table 12.1

1	2	3	4	5	6
What	How	When	Where	Why	Who
Definitory Hypothesis	ψ	Notation	Attention	Inquiry	Action
Oracle	Tiresias	Crossroads	Sphinx	Oedipus	Destiny

Table 12.1 includes clinical material that will employ the questions previously mentioned and their relations to functions and aspects of the Oedipus myth
(Oedipal Grid).

The patient arrives in the waiting room slightly late, talking on his cell phone.
Upon being invited to the consulting room by the analyst, he continues his phone
conversation while entering. He walks past the analyst as if the analyst were invisible. His eyes, marked by concern and somewhat troubled gestures, are fixed on a
distant point.

Simultaneously, he holds another cell phone in his other hand. Before ending the call, he lies down on the couch and, while turning off the first phone, checks the second one. He tells the person on the line, "I have to turn it off because I am entering a business meeting."

Aligning with Bion's perspective, our meeting, the analytic session is a "bad job." The patient seems disturbed by the analyst's presence, even though the analyst is merely performing their paid professional role and the patient attends the session voluntarily. Yet, this logical understanding seems to disappear as the patient, showing irritation, resorts to telling a lie to excuse the interruption of the session by a fact from his external life. Yet, in a way, this fabrication holds truth, as negotiations are inherent in the analytic process.

The analyst, with a "Good morning!" jokingly conveys an ironic undertone, subtly interrupts the patient's absorption in his phone.

The patient, highly intelligent and perceptive, grasps the subtlety and shows mild anxiety in responding, "Good morning." He explains,

Today, I've already made almost ten phone calls. Four of those calls averaged 24 minutes each. My last call was 22 minutes, according to my calculation… It took exactly 45 minutes to get here from my office, almost the equivalent of two calls. I was a bit late because idiot engineers have organized this city's traffic. Everyone knows the traffic lights should be synchronized, except for the Mayor and his team. I don't need to call his party; it's obvious.

The patient continues,

That's revolting! By the way, talking about the municipality, they built a field for the Pope to celebrate a mass, knowing that everything would go wrong in that place. It rained and the field became a swamp. What a waste of time and public money! However, don't be deceived; it was a fraud; the contractor prepared the ground to build a private residential condominium after.

While the patient voices numerous complaints, perhaps aimed at the analyst too, the analyst allows his imaginative and rational conjectures to emerge and navigate a path.

The analyst notes the patient's preoccupation with his phone upon arrival, as another manifestation of his generally detached demeanor. Attempting to engage more closely following the analyst's invitation into the session's reality, the patient briefly complains about the traffic before retreating. He navigates through topics such as technology, progress, the state, action, and freedom, with each concept prompting further inquiry. Amid these modern concerns, lies a deeper existential question: Is he truly living, or merely trying to survive? This distinction between existing and living presents a pivotal exploration.

In *Attention and Interpretation* (1970), Bion cites the poem, "The Rime of the Ancient Mariner," and elaborates, "The frightful fiend represents indifferently the quest for truth or the active defenses against it, depending on the vertex."[4] These vertices—of pursuing truth or evading it—are located in Grid's column 1, the Definitory Hypothesis, representing a "methodology of choice." column 2, represented by ψ, can be termed the "methodology of doubt."

For instance, from the vertex of truth, the previous clinical material illustrated a patient's struggle in making a choice between seeking truth through psychoanalysis (Definitory hypothesis), or employing defenses against truth (column 2, ψ).

In other words, a Definitory Hypothesis may simply pose a question: *WHAT is psychoanalysis*? Is it a place to explore one's unconscious? A setting where self-knowledge is sought? If this is the case, it might resemble visiting a place, a point, a space of the Oracle to pose questions. Therefore, the point reduces time to "now." Of course, we might hope otherwise, for the Oracle provided Oedipus with half-truths, effectively amounting to a clever deception.

Both the patient and the analyst may pose this question, seeing it as a beneficial inquiry. Yet, prior to engaging with psychoanalysis, any response merely outlines what psychoanalysis is not. Thus, our answers can only delineate its boundaries by stating what it does not encompass. For example, it is neither financial advice, marriage counseling, nor a means to foretell the future.

On the other hand, psychoanalysis explores a spectrum of possibilities and meanings. It lacks predetermined structures, focusing instead on a central inquiry: Truth. This cornerstone posits truth as a foundational element of our being, rendering life a meaningful path. Yet, this inquiry, akin to all potential constructs, suggests that definitive conclusions remain elusive. Truth is always in "dark deep waters."[5]

HOW, then, is psychoanalysis conducted? Before undergoing the emotional experience, psychoanalysis remains a mystery. Only through engaging in an analytic experience—a journey marked by both frustration and encounters with the unknown—does one begin to comprehend. Without this experience, there would be a tendency to move in the opposite direction of seeking truth, toward seeking a narrative to fill the gap. Within the Grid, the *Notation* (column 3) introduces a pivotal inquiry: WHEN did this entire narrative begin?

The foundational act of psychoanalysis is a manifestation of social autonomy, signifying a profound value deeply rooted in creative freedom. This statement encapsulates an ethical purpose. Drawing on Paul Ricoeur's philosophy, ethics involves the dynamics of engaging with a foreigner, highlighting the inherent strangeness stemming from the "not-me." This concept of "not-me" creates an empty space, a void, which manifests as a sense of loneliness, a theme prevalent in numerous ancient narratives.

Freud explored the theme of loneliness by revisiting the iconic biblical story of Moses in Egypt. He portrayed the Hebrew foreigner, "disguised" as an Egyptian prince, experiencing a profound moment of loneliness, leading to the revelation of his identity.

These narratives reveal a deep-seated philosophical unease, which in psychoanalysis, culminates in a specific metaphysical dimension: the individual's access to the truth about one's own narrative, as well as the truth of one's Oedipal configuration. This is not a philosophical truth, but rather truth as an ongoing search for improving humanity.

Moses and Oedipus,[6] both adopted by the queen of a foreign land, were unaware of their outsider status. Prompted by an encounter with a "not-me," they embarked on a quest for their origins, a journey that can be likened to a method of clarification or Notation. This approach aligns with the pivotal question: WHEN did their stories begin?

Humans are historical beings. Our past is an inherent component of our present. Psychoanalysis continually revisits and transforms our understanding of this link. Therefore, perceiving the past is not a static or irrefutable entity defying reflection. This reevaluation of our temporal perspective empowers individuals to explore their vicissitudes of truth, traversing both personal and collective historical landscapes.

In *On Arrogance* (1957), Bion *re-dimensions* the core inquiry of psychoanalysis from sexuality to an unreachable truth, applying the vertex of tragic ethics to reinterpret the Oedipus myth, highlighting the arrogance of the characters. He outlines a transition from Freud's dramatic ethics of avoiding sexual crimes and homicide to scenarios where arrogance, possibly spurred by hidden envy, fosters deceit, suicide, and destruction.

In *Attention and Interpretation* (1970), Bion revisits this theme through three Oedipal configurations: the symbiotic, where conservatism attempts to control the creativity; the parasitic, dominated by sterility and destruction; and the commensal, representing an agreement.

Bion, like Sophocles and Freud, searches for historical truth, acknowledging that the unattainable truth manifests through the creative and destructive process.

Let us now explore this theme through the Oedipus myth, focusing on the pivotal crossroads scene where Oedipus, unknowingly, seals his fate by killing his father, Laius.[7] The moment of Oedipus at the crossroads represents a state of potentiality; he is not yet a king or a patricide, highlighting the crucial act of choice and marking his transition from ignorance to awareness.

The pause, the brief moment between question and answer, encapsulates the essence of the crossroads. It represents a space of infinite potential, embodying both all roads and no roads simultaneously. It is akin to a deep breath taken before embarking on a journey or completing a transition, symbolizing the threshold between decision and action.

A person at a crossroads, undecided on a direction, occupies a unique in-between space, not fully on one path nor the other. This position transforms the crossroads into more than a symbol of death or paradox; it becomes a space for metaphor and creative action, the potent generators of complexity and richness in Life.

In my view, Bion's theory of transformations is rooted in his profound engagement with *complexity*, aimed at uncovering Truth at the core of psychoanalysis. This core features a crossroads where the act of playing a role blurs the line between being and not being that role. Similarly, a metaphor joins two terms in such a way that they simultaneously are and are not one another.

Another example of the complexity in Bion's ideas lies in experimenting various ways of time according to each type of transformation. Time, an essential feature of the crossroads, denotes the point of final decision between altering reality or evading it.

The starting point for envisioning these different modes of time are in the vicissitudes of Realization. These vicissitudes will determine the type of temporal experience, initially translated into a conception and, later, by a concept concerning time. The purpose of such an investigation is an Inquiry (column five), represented as the horizontal axis of the Grid at the fifth row, posing the question: WHY do those facts happen to a patient?

Through this inquiry, one may ultimately pose the question: WHO is the patient who seeks analysis? Who tells a dream? Who is the dreamer who dreams the dream? Who makes a lapse, a Freudian slip? Who undergoes a psychotic break? Who is coming to the session today? Conversely, who sits in the armchair as the analyst? Why does this person think he or she is qualified to define who a psychoanalyst is?

This individual, who claims to be a psychoanalyst, has certainly devoted considerable amount of time to training analysis, attending seminars, reading Freud's complete works, and studying hundreds of books on psychoanalysis and various other subjects. Yet, this extensive training and the credentials granted by recognized organizations do not guarantee a lasting desire and aspiration to practice analysis. What happens when one's desire to practice psychoanalysis fades away?

During extensive analytical training, when a candidate ponders, "Who am I?" can they truly find a clarifying answer? Engaging with a training analyst, who brings personal memories, desires, and Oedipal dynamics to the process and offers interpretations, still leaves the revelation of truth uncertain. Can anyone assure an affirmation such as: "Yes, you can be an analyst"?

Human singularity, according to the abstraction of the horizontal axis of the Grid (representing uses of elements), employs methods for expressing "judgements on the health-giving effect of the theory"[8] applicable across all psychic experiences. These experiences then evolve vertically, becoming progressively complex (representing growth).

This postulated approach introduces an alternative method for conceptualizing Bion's Grid, highlighting both its horizontal and vertical dimensions of meaning.

The Grid's first column, addressing the question "What?" as in, "What is psychoanalysis?" represents a selection process, similar to any choice, which inherently involves excluding other options.

In the second column (ψ), the omnipotence of the unconscious determines the decision-making process, aligning with the "How?" question, such as "How to conduct psychoanalysis?"

In the third column (Notation), the mind's hallmark of freedom of imagination leads to a method for historical clarification, corresponding to the question "When?" This notion of time opens the fourth column (Attention) to the question of space "Where?", which in turn advances to the fifth column (Inquiry), adopting the method of investigation: "Why?"

Ultimately, the sixth column (Action), a collective method, culminates with the final question "Who?" as the outcome of the preceding five methods, prompting inquiries such as "Who is the patient?"

In clinical material, one might employ the "servants" from Kipling's poem—What, How, When, Where, Why, Who—and, as Bion expanded, incorporate the "seventh servant"—Rest (leisure), representing a period of reflection. These elements provided knowledge derived from experiences and interactions with the unknown.

Imagine reaching a level of knowledge where we have all the questions necessary to progress towards becoming oneself. At this juncture, Bion's concept of *at-one-ment* might be applicable. This *becoming* could feel like a poetical awe, a multifaceted term, one aspect of which might be happiness. However, the symmetry between any mental state with singularity introduces difficulties, with frustration being the most frequent one.

For instance, one should think about an idea as something that brings happiness or as something that resonates with truth. The distinction between pursuing happiness as a goal and seeking truth raises a crucial question. For patients like those described, the core dilemma often revolves around the choice between living a life that is worth living and merely surviving.

In the search for happiness, a patient might falsify transient objects as permanent, since greed drives one toward eternal objects. This leads to a state of mind that may evolve into awe, but with a very different meaning. However, prior to greed, one must experience a sense of emptiness. This situation presents a paradox: the person who is fearful of facing emptiness creates an empty life. Here, the concept of symmetry, intrinsic to the complexity of the psychoanalytic object, becomes useful: greed is symmetric to happiness, as awe is symmetric to emptiness.

The patient's reliance on technology, driven by a fear of loss, links to a primitive, not modern, state of mind that remains present.

Situations that arouse feelings of awe, apprehension, and astonishment may evoke a sense of the majestic or sublime, akin to Hope, once experienced in encounters with the mother's mind-breast, the first object of pre-conception.

The concept of pre-conception centers on the perpetual, vague anticipation of an omnipotent object in *the future* that promises psychic gratification and elimination of a perceived sense of incompleteness. This enduring expectation, according to Bion, is anchored in the depths of the unconscious. However, integrating the concept of time into the timeless unconscious introduces controversy, or rather Complexity. Yet, this intricate idea paves the way for a seemingly paradoxical notion of *A Memoir of the Future.*

In every patient, this vague feeling is directed toward the analyst, harboring a hope that the analyst is in possession of *the* omnipotent interpretation capable of resolving all problems. This expectation hints at envisioning the future, intertwining emotional imagination, creativity, and thinking with language.

Keats's poem "On First Looking into Chapman's Homer" exemplifies awe and revelation, depicting the moment Keats discovers Homer through Chapman's translation. This moment is likened to Cortez's first view of the Pacific Ocean from the Serranía del Darién,[9] capturing a shared astonishment with "a wild surmise" among his crew.

Is a *wild surmise* akin to a wild thought?

"The Road Not Taken"[10] embodies the decision-making process, reflecting on the significance of choosing a path that might lead to the point of wild surmise. It also criticizes the notion of the self that emerges from these choices, emphasizing that the chosen path is ultimately less important than the decisive moment of choice at the crossroads of life.

Within ourselves, we may find a voice drawn to less traveled paths, yet hindered by doubt, uncertain about continuing and apprehensive about a potentially unchanged future.

Indeed, we will encounter paths that can make all the difference, those that loop back to the same, and ones that merely lead to other paths. Yet, above all, we face the centrality of the deep-seated dilemma at the crossroads: *the Oedipus complex*.

Notes

1   Numerous studies measuring radio spectrum usage have identified a significant portion of underutilized radio spectrum. To address this inefficiency, a shift toward more adaptable regulations through Dynamic Spectrum Access (DSA) has been suggested. The analysis of various facets of DSA systems, such as cooperative sensing, necessitates robust spatial models of spectrum utilization. Currently, the available models are narrowly focused, centering on specific aspects like propagation or shadowing correlation models. By adopting methodologies from spatial statistics, a more detailed application to spectrum modeling can be achieved. This involves using random fields and the semi-variogram to capture the spatial correlation of spectrum usage. Parameters derived from comprehensive real-life measurements across various wireless technologies have been extracted. These parameter sets provide a foundation for other researchers to apply this model across a spectrum of activities, from theoretical explorations to simulation-based research. This work was presented at the IEEE International Conference on Communications (ICC) in 2009.

2   W.R. Bion, *Transformations*, 1965, Karnac Books, p. 95.

3   "I keep six honest serving-men (They taught me all I knew); their names are What and Why and When, And How and Where and Who. I send them over land and sea, I send them east and west; but after they have worked for me, I give them all a Rest..." (Rest refers to the seventh servant). Rudyard Kipling.

4   W.R. Bion, *Attention and Interpretation*, 1970, Jason Aronson, p. 46.

5   J. Milton, *Paradise Lost*, III.

6   Marthe Robert, *From Oedipus to Moses: Freud's Jewish Identity*, 1976, translated by Ralph Manheim, Anchor Books, p. 229. This book examines how Freud's Jewish background and his understanding of the plight of European Jews manifested in his theory of psychoanalysis. An examination of Freud's private correspondence and personal dream records shows how Freud lived between the Jewish legacies of his father and the scientific, Christian culture of 19th century Vienna.

7 Unless we think of fate as predetermined by a higher power, pondering the debate be-tween free will and predestine. Yet, this debate is not the focus of our discussion.

8 W.R. Bion, *Transformations*, 1965, Karnac Books, p. 53. The term used by Bion as "health-giving effect" refers to Aristotle's similar notion in "Topics."

9 The Serranía del Darién, a mountain range on the Colombia-Panamá border within the Darién Gap, features Darién National Park in Panamá and Los Katíos National Park in Colombia. Its sparse population and remote accessibility, with the nearest town of 50,000 more than 12 hours away by road, highlight its isolation. Keats inaccurately placed it in Mexico, a notable error in his poetic depiction.

10 Robert Frost, *The Road Not Taken and Other Poems*, first published in 1915.

Chapter 13

Transformation in "O"

A Never-ending Transformation

This chapter delves further into the investigation of psychoanalytic transformation by the vertex of complexity, focusing on Bion's (1965) concept of "transformation in O." It explores the process of *how one becomes what one is*,[1] or the idea of becoming, in contrast to knowing.

> Transformation in K has, contrary to the common view, been less adequately expressed by mathematical formulation than by religious formulation. Both are defective when required to express growth, and therefore transformation, in O.[2]

Bion's "O" initially serves as an ideogram to address the epistemological needs arising from utilizing an *empty concept*, meaning a concept not saturated with meanings and open to experience. Moreover, it highlights the intrinsic limitations of psychoanalysis's core challenge: understanding the unconscious as a quantic concept through the ethical-aesthetical principles of uncertainty and infinity. This challenge is articulated through notions of truth, absolute truth, ultimate reality, and thought without a thinker (Bion, 1970, 1975, 1979).

In essence, "O," akin to "Onthos," signifies an unattainable origin while concurrently representing a dynamic process, as in "Opus," a work in progress. Both interpretations capture a core principle, illustrated as a never-ending wave, paralleled in science by the concept of a *soliton*.[3]

This framework acknowledges the unconscious as an "essence" governed by the *uncertainty principle of observation,* suggesting its exact nature and dynamics are elusive—the more we understand one aspect, the less we comprehend others. Furthermore, it introduces the *singularity principle*, advocating for an ongoing quest to reconcile the infinite aspects of human singularity with our finite existence.

"O" represents complexity, embodying an *ultimate difference* or *an unknowable ultimate reality.* It carries a wide range of associations, highlighting the relation between uncertainty and singularity encountered by psychoanalysts in the *analytical field.*

The concept of complexity redefines the analyst's *function* and *place* as one of ultimate difference—a realm of *impossibility.* This paradox, where the analyst's position as "the analyst" negates the actual process of analysis, underscores

DOI: 10.4324/9781003474128-14

Complexity's inherent logical contradictions. It suggests that psychoanalysis, akin to poetry, should be prepared to employ imagination to create a "second language" to conduct psychoanalysis. This approach emphasizes the necessity of innovation in the practice of psychoanalysis, paralleling the creative processes in art.

Bion's *Transformations* (1965) is notable for its embrace of complexity, rooted in intuition, a quality that often leads readers to find the book challenging.

Bion (1965, 1970, 1975) emphasizes a crucial condition for advancing psycho-analytic function of the analyst: building on Freud's propositions on attaining the state of sensorial deprivation, Bion advocates for an analytical mindset free from memory, desire, and the need for comprehension. These elements hinder the sen-sorial domain necessary for perceiving the psychoanalytic object. However, this introduces complexity, as complete sensorial deprivation is not only unachievable but also counterproductive to the analytic goal, given that alpha function (primarily symbolic) cannot exist without reverie (predominantly sensorial).

Bion's proposal to work without memory and desire does not aim at achieving a pure function but rather to maintain a critical reference that highlights the transition between different vertices, making *transference* possible. The analyst's function is to interpret, as their *countertransference* allows, from as many diverse vertices as possible to facilitate *analytical transformations*.

Exploring the analyst's *place* and *function* delves into the essence of complexity within the concept of "O," the point of ultimate difference. The relationship with "O" objectifies in the analytical act through the engagement of thinking of different vertices. The nature of the observed phenomena—be it neurosis, perversion, psy-chosis, dreams, parapraxes, myths, poetry, science, art, philosophy, or modernity—is secondary to the presence of a *limit* that reveals itself as an *enigma*, embodying complexity.

This limitation continuously compels the analyst to navigate toward this *enigma* through various vertices, indicating a pursuit for freedom of thought that fosters self-originality. This leads to considering transformation in "O" as an "original transformation," akin to the creative essence found in poetry and myth.

I think, labeling the process as "original" aligns with Bion's epistemological framework without diminishing its integrity. The term "original" not only high-lights its derivation from "O" as in O-rigin (Onthos)—presumably reflecting Bi-on's intent—but also encapsulates its development as in *Opus*, a work in progress akin to artistic process. This denotes an emotional experience of a new beginning.

Transformation in "O" is depicted as a process of bringing the analysand as close as possible to their true potential. According to Bion (1965), this process, termed K → O, prioritizes interpretive movement over hermeneutic or deterministic ap-proaches (Laplanche, 1993).[4] It is an endeavor to *translate enigmatic messages* beyond mere knowledge (K) toward a profound and authentic becoming ("O").

This translation is pivotal for psychological development. Interpreting is, in a sense, *deconstructing* what is already known, opening space-time for thoughts, thereby facilitating *new construction* of the subject as the essence of the analysand's task: K opens a future. *To interpret* is to uncover the essence of one's *Being* in the midst of historical evolution by means of differences of vertices.

These characteristics form a unique theory of the unconscious in Bion's model. The unconscious as *the origin of pre-conceptions*, which aims for psychic actualizations and shapes human structure through conceptions and concepts. This indicates that singularity arises from the impact of enigmatic conception of potentialities, surpassing the socio-historical existence of the subject and breaking into the totality of the real, valued as *forms of thought*. With an infinite array of thoughts, Bion's theory of pre-conception unveils a vast, complex domain for psychoanalysis.

Notes

1 *Ecce Homo: How One Becomes What One Is* is Nietzsche's last original work, written in 1888 but published posthumously in 1908. The book offers insight into his philosophical ideas and personal reflections on his life and works.
2 W.R. Bion, *Transformations*, 1965, Karnac Books, p. 156.
3 In mathematics and physics, a soliton is a non-linear, self-reinforcing, localized wave packet that is strongly stable. It preserves its shape while propagating freely at constant velocity and recovers it even after collisions with other such localized wave packets. Aleksandr S. Davydov, *Solitons in Molecular Systems*, Mathematics and its Applications (Series), Vol. 61 (2nd ed.), 1991, Kluwer Academic Publishers.
4 Laplanche distinguishes between two main interpretive perspectives: the deterministic, emphasizing Freud's view where the present is determined by a factual past, and the creative-hermeneutic, which seeks to ascribe meaning to a previously meaningless past. Laplanche critiques the binary between interpreting factual reality and subjective fantasy, proposing a third category: the "message." This concept focuses on the inherent meaning within the message, especially in the form of non-verbal sexual messages from adults to children, as a resolution to the antithesis.

Chapter 14

The Myth of Satan

An Ethical-Aesthetical Model of Transformation in "O"

Although I have previously discussed segments of this chapter in my book *A Lonesome Road*, I have decided to include it here to emphasize the significance of Milton's phrase "won from the void and formless infinite," as cited by Bion in *Transformations*.

Bion devoted significant attention to the complex relationship between language as a means of conveying aspects of truth or avoiding it. His fascination with the intricacies of various forms of language is evident across his body of work. In his book *Attention and Interpretation*, he pays particular attention to this theme, examining the use of languages in different disciplines. The final chapter of his book contrasts the Language of Achievement with the Language of Substitution.[1]

The complexity inherent in applying ethical-aesthetical principles of observation serves as a reminder that within every verbal being, there lies an *enigma* encapsulated within words. Psychoanalysis unveils this enigma through a synchronic landscape, where the aesthetic power of *myth* and *poetry,* linked with the ethics of thinking, aims to contain psychic pain.

Bion (1965) elucidated this landscape in psychoanalysis as a domain of transformations, marking the juncture where the complexities of various disciplines such as psychoanalysis, art, and mathematics intersect.

At the juncture where these vertices intersect, I (Chuster, 1997a, 2002, 2014, 2018) discuss one of the most tragic and eloquent myths in human history: the myth of Satan, as embodied in John Milton's *Paradise Lost*. The following discussion will focus specifically on its influence on Bion's concept of *transformation in "O"* (1965). Consequently, the discussion will not adopt a comprehensive approach to include the myriad folk and popular versions of the myth. The use of this myth serves as an example of row C in Bion's Grid, employed here to develop some ideas.

In *Paradise Lost*, the author, falling under the sortilege of the character initially intended for criticism (as did Cervantes in *Don Quixote* and Byron in *Don Juan*), subverts the traditional form of the myth. Instead of depicting a Christian and popular personification of Evil, he presents a hero who justifiably rebels against a tyrant—God. Empson[2] stated, "the reason why the poem is so good is that it makes God so bad ... the poem is wonderful because it is an awful

DOI: 10.4324/9781003474128-15

warning not against eating the apple but against worshipping that God." The poem reveals the authentic tragedy of humankind: Gods no longer reside where humans once sought them. They have left forever, leaving humans in solitude (Chuster 1997, 2018).

Contemporary critics acknowledged that a common error among several generations of scholars was their exclusive religious interpretation of the poem. Consequently, *Paradise Lost* was often considered as a profound discourse on "*the inscrutable ways of Divine Providence*" to "*assert Eternal Providence and justify the ways of God to Men.*" However, Robson[3] argues that Milton was essentially a heretic, challenging the Trinity, infant baptism, church-sanctioned marriage, the exclusivity of monogamy, and the belief in the soul's immortality. Milton perfectly fits the expression by the distinguished Brazilian poet Carlos Drummond de Andrade: "I am a man poor in beliefs and rich in doubts."

Milton was at the forefront of young writers and intellectuals who opposed Stuart's rule, an unyielding polemicist and pamphleteer, yearning for the "good old cause" of Cromwell's regime. Therefore, it is understandable to interpret Satan as a manifestation of Milton's skepticism toward the cultural beliefs and political system of his era. Furthermore, Satan, as portrayed by John Milton—a hero-villain with piercing, "*baleful eyes*"—as a compelling and fictional entity, transcends any religious or political allegories suggested by the poem's narrative.

Additionally, I propose an imaginative conjecture regarding Bion's identification with John Milton and his portrayal of Satan. All characters were *escaping* the confines of the Establishment to foster creativity.

The mystical elements represented in various descriptions of God as "*the Great Mystery, whose inscrutable ways can be comprehended only in the 'light' which is as yet inaccessible to men*" (an aspect some critics align with St. John of the Cross's reflections in *Ascent to Mount Carmel*), ought to be interpreted through the framework proposed by Bion (1970). He describes this as the *complex intuition of an unreachable truth*, defined by plurality, originality, and complexity, which serves as a focal point for both followers and opponents in a permanent confrontation.

From a socio-historical perspective, the unreachable truth discussed by John Milton remarkably anticipates modernity, marked by its defining trajectory of critique (targeting religion, morals, law, and politics), revolution (as an instrument for social change, and, in the Kantian sense, a fundamental methodological shift), and an allusion to the discovery of the dual infinities (the *cosmic* and the *psychological*). These elements precipitated a profound crisis in humanity's conceptual underpinnings, particularly those with an anthropocentric orientation. Consequently, the notion of a *fall*, perceived as a narcissistic wound to the Self, transforms modernity into a "diabolical project," and the character suffering this mythological descent becomes the "Great Satan" of Islamic fundamentalists and other religious and ultraconservative groups.

It can be posited that the tragic ethics depicted, representing humanity's quest for an unreachable truth in modernity, renders Satan as Milton's seminal creation, one that has spawned numerous literary descendants (Chuster, 1997).

The character of Satan finds a parallel in Byron's Don Juan, reflecting the rebellious spirit inherent in the use of poetic language. This figure acts as the earthly double, the corporeal and spiritual counterpart of Satan, embodying the *angel of freedom*.

For Baudelaire, Satan is depicted as *the fallen angel*, epitomizing the quintessential urban man. He descends into the city, adorned in elegant yet worn black attire, subtly marked by stains of wine, oil, and mud. At times provincial, at others the embodiment of the avant-garde, he makes the essence of modernity manifest through close associations with machinery, leisure, and sexuality.

Apollinaire portrays him as a city tramp, a *poor devil* wandering lost and alone among the crowd, yet facing the multitude with his frail and awkward stature. He criticizes those who arrogantly underestimate him, perceiving him as naive and attempting to exploit him. Yet, in reality, he is vulnerable and sensitive to all that is human; he embodies the figure portrayed by Chaplin in films: a creature brimming with energy, simultaneously a clown and a magician, a passionate, anonymous man, bewildered by the cruelty of those who proclaim to speak in the name of God. These facets, many of them paradoxical, invite examination through a lens of complexity, one of whose tenets includes the Uncertainty principle, as articulated by Keats and further emphasized by Bion as *negative capability*.[4]

Therefore, the myth of Satan facilitates an exploration, from the vertex of the search for truth as highlighted by Bion, across three dimensions of human experience: the *socio-historical vertex* (charting the vicissitudes of humanity into modernity); secondly, the realm of dream-like language observed and utilized by psychoanalysis, and thirdly, as a domain of complexity.

In another sense, we might argue that psychoanalysis is inherently modern. In addition, psychoanalysis can be considered *the voice of human complexity*. This leads to the question: to what extent does the analytical process enable the analysand to attune to modernity? Could modernity be characterized as the enhancement of critical and reflective capacities to make responsible decisions, facilitated by properly elaborating the confrontation between finitude and infinitude?

Simultaneously, it is necessary to forge a psychoanalytic link that could elucidate the psychotic aspect of the personality (Bion, 1956) while mitigating the envious inhibition of growth-producing good objects.[5] This task, I think, cannot be achieved without employing transformations through a non-linear critique, found within a non-linear thinking space, such as Hilbert space.

This type of critique, as featured in *Transformations* (Bion, 1965), is further exemplified in two of Bion's works, *The Grid* (1963) and the *Advanced Grid* (1970). Both serve as reminders of the application that analysts should make of negative capability.

To this understanding, I introduced the concept of a *Negative Grid* (Chuster, 1999, 2002, 2014, 2018), clarifying that the Negative Grid holds a distinct meaning from negative capability. The Negative Grid aims to trace the destructive aspects of the personality as it grapples with the principles of infinity and uncertainty in creation and meanings, and their clash with human finitude. This perpetual conflict proves unbearable to the psychotic component of the personality.

The ethical-aesthetic principles of infinity and uncertainty originate from the scientific discoveries of cosmic infinity by mathematics and psychological infinity by psychoanalysis.

These discoveries unveiled a new horizon that was unimaginable to pagan antiquity, and even less so to the Christian Middle Ages. For instance, Dante's Universe was finite, enabling him to map Hell, Purgatory, and Heaven. In this limited world, man was eternal, destined to live forever, whether in damnation or in bliss. In stark contrast, the modern man inhabits an infinite universe yet is doomed to vanish forever. This constitutes the radical divergence between the modern and the medieval worlds. Regardless of our actions, our existence is unavoidably tragic and, therefore, *satanic*. We roam a universe where black holes, as Hawking[6] demonstrated in astrophysics, confirm the reality of infinity—not only in the realm of imagination but also, as Cantor and Pascal had previously shown, within the domains of writing and mathematical thought, as a concrete, determinable, feasible reality.

It seems pertinent here to recall Bion's citation of Pascal at the conclusion of *Transformations*: "*Le silence des ces espaces infinis m'effraie*" (1965), reflecting a profound awareness of the vast emotions and imperfect thoughts that govern our human nature.

Notes

1 W.R. Bion (1970). *Attention and Interpretation*. Tavistock. (Re-printed Karnac, 1984.), p. 126.

2 William Empson, *Milton's God*, 1979, Bloomsbury Publishing.

3 W.W. Robson, "Paradise Lost: Changing Interpretation and Controversy," a chapter in *The New Pelican Guide to English Literature, Vol. 3: From Donne to Marvell*, edited by Boris Ford, 1982, Penguin Books Ltd.

4 W.R. Bion, *Attention and Interpretation*, 1970, Rowman & Littlefield Publishers Inc., p. 125.

5 W.R. Bion, *Attention and Interpretation*, 1970, Rowman & Littlefield Publishers Inc., p. 129.

6 In the introduction to Stephen Hawking's *A Brief History of Time* (1988), Carl Sagan writes, "This is also a book about God... or perhaps about the absence of God... a universe with no edge in space, no beginning or end in time, and nothing for a Creator to do."

Chapter 15

Transformations in Hallucinosis

An Utmost Clinical Challenge

Numerous instances of transformation in hallucinosis occur and can be observed in individuals who rigidly adhere to political or religious beliefs, becoming impervious to dissent and ideological debates. It is plausible to suspect that such individuals may be experiencing a confusional state of mind, consequently resulting in significant anxiety that gives rise to dogmatic thinking.

These beliefs remain unaltered even when confronted with compelling evidence from reality. Some quickly take offense at any confrontation with doubt, indicating that the dimension to which they adhere employs a moralistic discourse. This discourse does not manifest openly; rather, it is silent, blind, and deaf, operating through a *Language of Substitution*.[1]

Nevertheless, a *Language of Substitution* is capable of communicating with others; therefore, it would find an audience, inevitably leading to the emergence of contradictions.

Contradictions frequently exemplify the *minus K link*, especially if they are tinged with colors of arrogance, certainty, and violence. In their discourse, the term "conspiracy" frequently appears, symbolizing the rupture of commensal links within the Oedipal configuration, transforming them into adversaries embattled against one another under the auspices of a sort of God or deity.

In other words, when the Oedipal pre-conception (realized, for instance, as an integrated triangle of father, mother, and son, which primarily represents the three-dimensional nature of the human mind) fails to connect with proper objects, the tragedy of a vanished "deity" emerges. Should attempts to reinstate this "deity" prove ineffective, they invariably recur in a manner that disrupts the Oedipal links.

These individuals interpret any form of disagreement or contradiction as a personal offense, reacting with intense anger as though under attack. Their guiding principle is, "If you are not with me, you are against me." This perspective on reality precludes any form of discussion or inquiry into truth, as truth has become not a universal concept but a possession of a specific group. They consider themselves sole proprietors of truth, privy to revelations not accessible to others. Those who challenge their views are labeled as "infidels." Their behavior mirrors that of the Taliban sect, who regard themselves as the sole bearers of purity and truth, while viewing dissenters as deceivers and tricksters.

DOI: 10.4324/9781003474128-16

A humorous anecdote may help to shed light on this situation. A man in a psychiatric hospital was deemed psychotic for believing he was an ear of corn. After being treated with appropriate medication, he acknowledged that he was not, in fact, an ear of corn. The psychiatrist, considering him reconnected with reality, decided he could be discharged. Upon leaving the hospital, however, the sight of a chicken filled him with dread, as he perceived the chicken's gaze as "hostile." Hurriedly, he returned to the hospital seeking assistance. Puzzled by his return, the psychiatrist inquired why he came back, given his understanding that he was a person, not an ear of corn. The patient replied, "Yes, I know I'm not an ear of corn. But does the chicken know that?"

Let us imagine their dialogue continues further. The psychiatrist suggests that the chicken likely knows nothing, as chickens are incapable of thought. The patient replies, "You're trying to deceive me." The psychiatrist maintains his stance, arguing it is a matter of common sense. The patient responds, "No, no, you're trying to humiliate me. Do you believe your ideas are superior to mine?" In this exchange, each response is met with its opposite. The patient demonstrates an unusual application of common sense, reminiscent of a politician who interprets jeers as cheers. The interaction becomes a perpetual cycle. It highlights the cruelty of the superego and the rivalry with "O," alongside the employment of lies and the attempt to argue that these falsehoods prove that lies are superior to truth.

Imagine now an individual who perceives and conducts themselves as if they were a deity, yet masks this mindset with a language that shows little concern for the outcomes. Their speech is devoid of substantive proposals, laden with generalizations like "they," "the elites," "the middle class," "the people," "the poor," etc. These generalizations both characterize and unveil the presence of beta elements. They often convey perceptions of broad qualities but with a diminished affective tone, obscuring the significance of those words. Therefore, they are akin to a bodily experience that is challenging to identify.

For instance, when prompted to specify what is meant by generalizations such as "the elite" or "the people," the speaker merely alters their tone of voice to a more formal register, ignores the question, diverges onto unrelated topics, provides no direct answer, and moves away from the context of the ongoing dialogue. Should someone challenge or contradict the speaker's narrative, that challenger is labeled a Bigot. They have a stream of dead words, emblematic of the Party of Dead—the totalitarian party.

Like all gods masquerading as humans, they neither possess nor require any real power. All they need are institutions that glorify their image and utilize funds to amplify their message. Their presence is akin to a divine phantasm. Yet, their ultimate role is to deceive humans. Their fate is irrevocably tied to the employment of Lies, regardless of the consequences.

This situation reminds the story from the Mahabharata, where the god Krishna, disguised as the charioteer of the hero Arjuna, attempts to convince him by advocating for war with arguments that could lead the hero to his death or to the killing of relatives and friends. In such a situation, it becomes impossible to reconcile truth and history. Consequently, Arjuna refuses to fight, discarding his weapons, leading to the god's disappearance forever.

The god's vanishing creates a space that expands as the human disguise (falsehoods and lies) is discarded. What lingers between the two realms is the corporeal manifestation of the deity incarnate: the god remains present in his very absence. Yet, confining his existence to an image painted on screens or as tattoos in the skin, experienced through mantras and prayers, devoid of the once sacred "body to body" communion. Without the divide between gods and humans, neither truth nor history could find a place—only the divine form would persist. Hence, when someone adopts the mantle of godliness, he or she must resort to employ the unspoken, empty words that suggest a presence at once absent and incomplete. Every unvoiced subject nurtures the hope for a divine link. The deity disappears with the utterance of truth. For gods, sincerity is forbidden.

The individual assuming the role of god is aware that he is not truly a deity, yet what he or others understand is of little consequence; his assertions cannot be challenged in matters of omnipotence. He declares, "That is all"—possessing a form of absolute knowledge that bears no dissension, yet it also cannot be articulated. Consider the scenario where he admits the truth, acknowledging he is not a god; the deception he has perpetuated for years could lead to his imprisonment.

This scenario exemplifies the domain that psychoanalysts explore: the vast territory of Lies and their derivatives. This realm is adeptly navigated by various criminals, including rapists, thieves, murderers, racketeers, drug dealers, and fraudulent politicians.

Transformation in Hallucinosis eradicates knowledge associated with uncertainty. Through the phenomenology of projective identification, it fosters elitist thought processes. Such ideas aim to establish moral superiority over all individuals outside the specific group, be it a society, party, or nation. Those not included in this exclusive circle are deemed misguided and errant.

Symmetric and ethical-aesthetic interpretations formulated in these situations evoke a dream-like possibility. On one side, there is the omnipotence of a silent god; on the other, the helplessness of a contemptible human who refuses to listen. Both are enveloped in blindness.

A patient of this nature may exhibit sadistic tendencies if the circumstances permit. Typically, though, they opt for a tyrannical stance toward the analyst, mocking them inwardly while outwardly maintaining a facade of politeness and gentleness. The disparagements are often subtle, accompanying the patient's reactions to the analyst's interpretations. They habitually respond to accurate interpretations with a "What?" as if they had not heard it or as though the analyst was speaking in a foreign tongue.

One can observe another instance of this ambiguous discourse in a female patient who identifies as a "communist" and supports this ideological stance by claiming her "political teachers" were prominent leaders she interacted with, thanks to her father, an influential politician. She references these leaders without any historical consideration, neglecting to acknowledge that she was a very young child (four to six years old) at the time, incapable of engaging in intellectual discussions with these elder statesmen. While she might have been present during their visits to her father's home, the assertion that she exchanged ideas with these political figures is, at best, a fairy tale. Yet, the veracity of her claims may not be as significant as appreciating the notion of being in proximity to a deity masquerading as a human. This situation illuminates the tacit rules governing the relationship she describes.

The patient makes no secret of her perceived superiority due to her "personal inspirations from great teachers." Leveraging the political power of her father through murky and unethical means, she secures million-dollar contracts for her work with the Government and resides in one of the city's most affluent neighborhoods. Yet, she expresses indignation toward the "elite" and the "upper middle class," criticizing their reluctance to share "space" with the impoverished (echoing the rhetoric of a demagogic leader, despite her exclusive travel in business class). She employs a moralistic logic that positions her above others, selectively acknowledging only facts that serve her interests. This intense primitive splitting—tearing the original links apart—is reconciled through transformations in hallucinosis.

This patient experienced trauma immediately following birth, as her mother suffered from post-partum psychosis, from which she never fully recovered. In the aforementioned encounters with prominent politicians, her mother was never present. She concealed her sense of void with a facade of omnipotence.

The sense of incompleteness always presents an opportunity for exploration. This possibility for inquiry depends on attributes that support the existence of the knowledge (K) link. The commitment to sincerity is essential in building trust, which, in turn, should cultivate further sincerity. The logic forms a circular pattern, where the circle's diameter becomes psychic intimacy.

Freud emphasized that all educational and ethical values in psychoanalysis rest on the practice of sincerity. This principle is central to the analytic relationship. Some patients are unaware that their feelings of terror, which manifest in associations as "hauntings," persist as long as they remain mere spectators of their lives, stuck in a perpetual state of fight or flight rather than taking action. Terror dissipates when the patient acknowledges the haunting feelings as their own, marking the beginning of a transformation into a new being. The shift occurs from spectator to protagonist, embarking on a journey of self-discovery. Through the mirror of language, new modes of thought and action are unveiled.

A patient noted improvement in his relationship with his girlfriend, attributing the progress to analysis. He shared a dream in which he had a singular image of being attacked by a vampire. He offered no further associations, only describing an intense feeling of terror experienced during the dream. The analyst aspired to "dream" the patient's dream, interpreting that a transformation in "O" might symbolically resemble the vampire that does not see its reflection in a mirror. This led to offering the patient two introspective questions: "Where is everything you ever knew about yourself?" and "Why is there no language that reflects who you are?"

The vampire, a character frequently depicted in films, periodically receives updated portrayals. Bram Stoker's tale acquires sophisticated nuances with advancements in technology. As with many literary figures, fresh interpretations emerge as film technology evolves. Yet, despite technological enhancements rendering scenes more aesthetically realistic, the underlying sense of fear neither intensifies nor lessens.

Consider an analogy that juxtaposes the analytical process with the transition from cinema to theater. This comparison highlights distinct experiential outcomes: cinema makes us dream, whereas theater prompts awakening. By analogy, the analytical process, akin to theater, makes contact with the dream, awakening the patient. In doing so, it transforms the dream, thereby facilitating the emergence of new dreams.

Theater has the power to extract us from the dream world by making the absence of truth accessible. It achieves this through the actor's presence, which introduces the dimension of absence. When a patient assumes the role of their missing objects and failures, they transition from a passive observer of their life to an active participant, marking a profound shift in their engagement with both their internal and external worlds.

The space in the scene between the actor and the spectator is akin to the space between various dualities such as container and contained, male and female. Within this space lies the origin of ethics and the sustenance required for the ethical Self's vitality. It is here that the silent challenge of the not-me surfaces, calling for respect, compassion, and understanding without judgement, thereby nurturing our dedicated responsibility as analysts. The obliteration of this space occurs when projective identification intensifies.

For example, a female patient challenges the analyst by stating he cannot comprehend her deeply due to gender differences, emphasizing with certainty and disdain that "a man" will inevitably face issues with women. The analyst identifies the generalization of conflict with women as a disguise, masking a deeper issue related to women's struggle to exist as women. This struggle seldom anchors in a fixed image of a mother, arresting their development since childhood, leading them to adopt a maternal role as a cover, making it difficult to move beyond this persona. However, they may take on the maternal role, they cannot fully embrace it.

This struggle may originate from the conflictual mother/daughter relationship, characterized by the intensity of projective identification that tends to erase individual differences. The more intense the projective identification, the more challenging it becomes for a daughter to embody roles such as wife and mother, despite her desire for these roles. Projective identification narrows the space for individuality and depletes the wellspring of aesthetic and ethical values, leading to a mutual expectation of complicity between mother and daughter, which restricts freedom. This lack of freedom may manifest in a tendency to think about death, evident in the patient's daily destructive activities. These behaviors impair her capacity to feel emotions and compel her to seek sensuality in physical activities.

What the patient perhaps implies by suggesting that the analyst, being a man, could not understand her as a woman is that the analyst would not be her accomplice. Thus, the *man* becomes the container for her destructive hatred, the evil eye.

The analytic process for this patient functions as a *scene* for generating new object representations through facilitating a dialogue between a man and a woman on another level. This dialogue allows for the emergence of representations beyond the maternal, and allows the man to be more than just a defender against the woman's complaints of dissatisfaction. This language captures the singularity of the case and the frustrating encounter with an object capable of integrating primitive elements (providing alpha function), highlighting the transformative potential of the analytic process.

The analytical scene enables the separation of the woman from the maternal role, transforming the patient from a passive spectator into an active participant, the actress capable of performing her role as a woman, thereby capable of creativity in life.

The man versus woman drama unfolds within the tragic dimension of an unknown *truth*, a topic central to analysis. This truth does not emerge through the assertion of dominance; it is not the province of either but manifests in their encounter, devoid of power struggle.

Several years ago, during an Olympic game, I observed a player stepping out of his role as a "player/actor" to angrily demand applause and support from the audience. In that moment, he ceased to be a player, focusing instead on dictating the spectators' role. This shift led to an immediate decline in his performance, suggesting a possible alignment with the audience's anxieties, thus amplifying his fear of failure. This underscores a crucial insight for an athlete during the most challenging moments: the importance of enjoying the game over perceiving the situation as a matter of life and death. Enjoying the game aligns performance with training, where discipline safeguards the athlete.

Drawing on this analogy, the analyst must cultivate "leisure" within sessions, setting aside the pressures from the patient to offer interpretations. Similarly, maintaining leisure in personal life—particularly, leisure of high quality—is essential for the effective performance of the analyst.

Actors in ancient Greek theater often experienced a state of mind akin to divine possession before entering the scene, which could enable them to deliver forewarnings. This state was not about prophesying in the literal sense, but rather it resembled an "apprehended memory of the future." The intensity of this possession was thought to correlate with the quality of the performance, suggesting a deep connection between the actor's mental state and their ability to convey the play's message effectively.

In sports, maintaining "concentration" before competitions is crucial. An Olympic team's focus was disrupted when a technical crew member brought up a personal issue, leading to emotional involvement and debate among the athletes. This shift from game preparation to philosophical discussions on the problem caused the team to enter the game unprepared, fostering a fear of loss. Unable to stay in their player role, they made numerous mistakes and ultimately lost the game. They had, in essence, embodied a loser.

Might the individual fear encountering danger during a session, such as witnessing a disturbing scene leading him to the verge of a breakdown? Alternatively, a breakup or divorce? Could a breakthrough be the next outcome, witnessing a nodal point where the individual encounters their inner "deity"?

This encounter establishes a confrontation between the disintegrative and integrative forces, signaling a pivotal moment to leave the gods behind. We must part ways with them to carry on with our own lives, relying solely on our humanity without the need for sacrifice. We should not be like Prometheus, Palinurus, or Christ. We should embrace our own path.

This divergence from the divine is analogously evident in the period when the ancient Greeks transitioned from religious rites at the altar to theatrical performances on the stage, signifying a departure from a divine-centered Renaissance to a focus on the resurgence of the Human Self.

This transition, from altar to stage in the sixth century BC, marked a significant cultural shift characterized by unprecedented creativity across philosophy and the arts. This period of enlightenment, reverberates with vitality into the present. The organized family of Olympus, which had once defeated Chronos' family, was defeated on stage by the family of philosophers and poets. Perhaps stage fright has its origins in this dynamic.

Defeating the gods ensures our humanity. Their divine presence diminishes as they retreat, yet not merely through distance or absence. They do not leave; they become absent from within.

Perhaps the gods vanish when sacrifices cease to maintain their presence: no sacrifice, no god. Humans have turned to writing, calculating, legislating, and analyzing. This should be recognized as the genuine story. As their presence fades, the truth of any story becomes uncertain.

The foundational myth of psychoanalysis is deeply rooted in Sophocles' plays, particularly in "Oedipus." This narrative originates from an archaic separation between the audience and the actors, a *Caesura* embodied in the concept of the *scene*, which also represents the separation between actor and chorus.[2]

What is the significance of the caesura between the actor and the chorus, and what was crucial before their separation? It can be noted that there existed a ritualistic group, followers of a highly revered god: Dionysus. This deity, known as the triune (three-in-one) figure, had his principal sanctuary in Ephesus. The devotees, referred to as Mystics, performed rituals that continue to exert an influence on contemporary Christian practices.

Initially, the Dionysian cult involved the ritual sacrifice of an animal, which was dismembered in a manner reflecting the number of participants. This act symbolized Dionysus's dismemberment by the Titans, highlighting his suffering. The Bacchantes' ritual aimed at reassembling Dionysus, symbolizing communal unity through the reconstitution of the god. This mirrors the Communion ritual, where each participant embodies a fragment of the divine, achieving unity through the shared experience. As with any ritual, this restoration of the deity is destined for indefinite repetition, thereby providing participants with a sense of eternal reunion with the divine.

In theater, with the appearance of the actor, the deity vanishes forever, unable to instill terror any longer, since the actor, through dialogue and play, eradicates the fear of the ghost. Similarly, in the analytic scene, reaching the *language of achievement* represents the discovery of a language that effectively communicates for both participants, resulting in the disappearance of "ghosts." This transition marks the process of becoming—*transformation in "O."*

This transformation in "O" sustains the impossibility of memory and knowledge, indicating that no memory or desire can facilitate this transformation—only a continuous movement toward becoming. The analyst embodies the void at the center of the analytical scene. The void representing a split from the original oneness, "O," symbolically echoed by a "chorus" of ideas. Through analytical work, the perception of an absence is made possible, introducing a third dimension that awakens the spectator. This awakening, though not always pleasant, signifies the emergence of something new.

Notes

1 W.R. Bion, *Attention and Interpretation*, 1970, Rowman & Littlefield Publishers Inc., p. 126.
2 The chorus is always present at the Greek Theater as a structure symbolizing a separation, a caesura.

Chapter 16

Always "O"

Ontology and Epistemology

"O" signifies *Onthos (origin)*, as found in ontology, and concurrently represents *Opus*, indicating "*work in progress*." These notions encapsulate epistemological facets of Bion's concept of "O." In essence, an origin is continuously at work. Given its constant evolution, it remains elusive, never to be fully captured. This ineffability can only be partially observed.

James Joyce, in *Finnegan's Wake*, employed the phrase "*work in progress*" to define an open model text—a text that invites endless interpretation from end to beginning. This concept introduces a circularity of language, reflecting an ever-evolving narrative structure that defies conventional linear reading, embodying a text in perpetual motion.

One might argue the necessity of pinpointing a "*caesura*" in this text, a pause of an internal nature. The selection of a *caesura* remains inherently subjective, decided upon by the reader. In psychoanalytic practice, either the psychoanalyst or the patient may initiate it. Yet, its appearance unveils a "*caesura of speculation*," the pure text, the anti-rhythm suspension that establishes unforeseen continuities within the expanse of the imagination.

One may view the "*work in progress*" as the forefront of "*restless thinking*" regarding a certain reality, where we might encounter a *thought without a thinker*,[1] possibly a *stray thought*, or a *thought with the owner's name and address upon it*, available for temporary adoption and subsequent return. If we are fortunate and genius-minded, we might encounter a *wild thought*, heralding a rare epistemological moment that decisively slices through history, demarcating a "before" and "after" the thought, which one may call *a road not taken*.

"O" embodies the Greek term *Ergon*, denoting both the productive work and the work product itself, with these two aspects in dialogue, aiming toward *Energeia*—the self-renewing *dynamism* (movement). The etymology of *Werk* in German and "*Work*" in English retains this Greek root: "*erg*."[2]

Notably, the word "*work*" lacks a Latin counterpart, deriving instead from *tripalium*, a term denoting a three-pronged whip employed by Roman overseers to coerce enslaved individuals into labor. The framework proposed by Bion, it bears repeating, advocates for an open system.

DOI: 10.4324/9781003474128-17

The foundation for grasping the concept of open systems is rooted in Kurt Gödel's theorem, which posits an irreparable rupture within any axiomatic system, allowing the formulation of theory and logic of open systems.

Gödel built upon Cantor's assertion that every set is essentially infinite. In light of this indeterminacy, Gödel juxtaposed two sets to demonstrate that within their collective propositions lie points of incompleteness and undecidability regarding their origin. This implies that within every relationship, there exists a moment where ownership cannot be definitively assigned. Does it pertain to the patient or the analyst? The patient or the family? The family or society? The mother or the child? The father or the mother?

One may discover a practical application of Gödel's theorem through the liar paradox, exemplified by the statement, "This sentence is false." The sentence cannot be true (since it declares itself false) nor false (as it would then be true). A Gödel sentence G within theory T echoes the liar's paradox but alters its provability: G states, "G is not provable in theory T." The examination of G's truth and provability serves as a formalized inquiry into the liar sentence's veracity.

It is not possible to equate "not demonstrable" with "false" in Gödel's framework, as the statement "Q is the Gödel number of a false formula" cannot be represented by a linear logic formulation. This principle underscores Tarski's theorem of indefinability, which Gödel independently discovered while developing his incompleteness theorem.

Werner Heisenberg drew upon Gödel's concepts in formulating his Uncertainty Principle, applying it to observational acts, thus enabling the emergence of complex object in contrast to simple object. Consequently, he introduced an epistemological division in scientific thought, delineating a distinct "before" and "after" his principle.

To illuminate the concept of the undecidable paradox, let us consider the famous paradox of the barber of Seville. The barber displayed a sign at his shop's entrance, which stated: "I only shave those who do not shave themselves." This raises the question: Who shaves the barber? This question creates a spiral of paradoxes. If the barber shaves himself, yet he shaves only those who do not shave themselves, then he should not shave himself. However, because he does not shave himself and shaves everyone else who does not, he paradoxically ends up shaving himself.

It is crucial to note that, from a mathematical perspective, the barber paradox is untenable due to the inherent contradiction in the barber's existence. Therefore, logically, either Seville does not exist or such a barber cannot reside there, illustrating the impossibility of such a contradictory scenario in reality.

Another instance of paradox is highlighted in the renowned *Star Trek* TV series. Surrounded by androids demanding a secret for his survival, Mr. Spock[3] states, "I will tell you the truth, but do not believe me for I am a liar." This presents the androids with a paradox that they are unable to resolve, ultimately leading to their malfunction.

This scenario illustrates the intuitionism[4] principles developed by mathematicians Brouwer and Heyting. They argued that if a proposition is true, its negation can also be true, introducing the concept of *a third* beyond the traditional binary of Aristotle's logic. This logic, comprehensible only to humans, echoes the Oedipus complex: if I am neither my father nor my mother, I still exist, embodying aspects of both within me.

Prior to the establishment of this epistemological approach, the notion of complexity was confined to everyday language. Engaging with a complex object entails grappling not only with quantities of units and interactions beyond straightforward calculation but also with elements of uncertainty, indeterminacy, randomness, chaos, and chance.

Complexity partially intersects with the uncertainty that stems from the limitations in our comprehension of phenomena. Consequently, knowledge is not merely a collection of facts we possess but rather a target of our ongoing pursuit. It resides in the potential of what we aim to discover in the future.

In psychoanalytic practice, knowledge is situated within the context of today's session, rather than being a continuation of previous ones. This approach eschews the formal logic that suggests a linear progression from one session to the next. These past sessions, though not false as logical propositions, are false or irrelevant as knowledge. It is crucial to recognize this paradoxical nature of psychoanalytic knowledge: it is anchored in the present session, yet it maintains the perspective of future sessions. This perspective forms a penumbra—a shadowy outline of future possibilities. It is a memoir of the future.

In poetical terms, it signifies that knowledge emerges during transition, such as dawn or dusk, where light and shadow intermingle, creating a realm of undecidable propositions that link two distinct phases. Is it the light of day, or the darkness of night? Here, the third state is a caesura.

This analogy to the twilight hours underscores that knowledge is not merely a beacon of light. In the ambiguous light of dawn or dusk, it becomes necessary to engage our imagination to navigate the gaps, the uncertainties. Explanations, in their clarity, often prevent us from capturing the essence of our inquiries, proving too definitive for the nuanced realms we explore.

The obscuring influence of these *explanations* finds resonance in Freud's correspondence with Lou Andreas-Salome, highlighting the necessity of "…casting a beam of intense darkness so that something which had been hitherto obscured by the glare of the illumination can glitter all the more in the darkness."[5]

A fundamental interchange exists between presence and absence. Nietzsche, in *Thus Spoke Zarathustra*, suggests that the day emerges not merely against the backdrop of night but through the possibility of the absence of night. Thereby, dawn and dusk surpass mere linguistic constructs; they also emerge as natural phenomena, embodying a form of chaos.

Learning can originate from both necessity and passion. Psychoanalysts, akin to pianists mastering scales either through technical discipline or through a love for music, may enhance their practice via rigorous study or profound passion for psychoanalysis, striving to advance their skills through experience. This path demands embracing the humility of our finite comprehension, presenting a choice between strict adherences to established rules for accuracy where all one can do are movements of approximations to an evanescent phenomenon. This pivotal choice probes the essence of our professional and personal lives as a real complexity. However, complexity provides us with a future.

Notes

1 W.R. Bion, *Taming Wild Thoughts*, 1997, Karnac Books, p. 27.
2 The CGS unit of work or energy. One erg is equivalent to 10^{-7} joule.
3 Leonard Simon Nimoy, the acclaimed actor, was born in Boston, Massachusetts, to Dora (Spinner) and Max Nimoy, who owned a barbershop. His parents were Ukrainian Jewish immigrants. Growing up in a tenement and performing in community theaters from the age of eight, Nimoy's Hollywood debut came at 20 with a minor role in *Queen for a Day* (1951).
4 L.E.J. Brouwer, states: "First Act of Intuitionism Completely separating mathematics from mathematical language and hence from the phenomenon of language described by theoretical logic, recognizing that intuitionistic mathematics is an essentially language less activity of the mind having its origins in the perception of a move of time. This perception of a move of time may be described as the falling apart of a life moment into two distinct things, one of which gives way to the other, but is retained by memory. If the twoity thus born, is divested of all quality, it passes into the empty form of the common substratum of all twoity. And it is this common substratum, this empty form, which is the basic intuition of mathematics." Brouwer's *Cambridge Lectures on Intuitionism*, 1981, edited by D. Van Dalen, Cambridge University Press, New York, pp. 4–5.
5 Ernst Pfeiffer (ed.), *Sigmund Freud and Lou Andreas-Salome Letters*, 1985, W. W. Norton and Company, p. 11.

Bibliography

Bion, W.R. (1956) Differentiation of the Psychotic and Non-psychotic Personalities. In *Second Thoughts* (pp. 43–64). Heinemann, London, 1967.

Bion, W.R. (1957) On Arrogance. In *Second Thoughts*. Jason Aronson Inc., Northvale, 1967.

Bion, W.R. (1962a) A Theory of Thinking. In: *Second Thoughts: Selected Papers on Psychoanalysis* (pp. 110–119). Heinemann, London, 1967.

Bion, W. R. (1962b). Learning from Experience. London: Heinemann. (Re-printed London: Karnac, 1984.) p. 70.

Bion, W.R. (1963) *Elementos de Psicanálise*. Zahar, Rio de Janeiro.

Bion, W.R. (1965) *Transformações*. Imago, Rio de Janeiro.

Bion, W.R. (1967). Notes on memory and desire. In: *Cogitations* (pp. 380–385). Karnac, London.

Bion, W.R. (1970) *Attention and Interpretation*. Tavistock, London. (Re-printed Karnac, 1984.)

Bion, W.R. (1975) *The Grid and Caesura*. Imago, Rio de Janeiro.

Bion, W. R. (1976). Clinical Seminars and Four Papers. Oxford: Fleetwood Press, 1987.

Bion, W.R. (1977a) *Two Papers: The Grid and Caesura*, ed. J. Salomao. Rio de Janeiro: Imago Editora. (Revised edition Karnac, 1989.)

Bion, W. R. (1977b). Seven servants. New York: Jason Aronson.

Bion, W.R. (1979) *A Memoir of the Future, Book III: The Dawn of Oblivion*. Clunie Press, Perthshire. (Also in *A Memoir of the Future, Books 1–3*. Karnac, 1991.)

Bion, W.R. (1994) *W.R. Bion: Clinical Seminars and Other Works*. Karnac, London.

Castoriadis, C. (1997) *World in Fragments: Writings on Politics, Society, Psychoanalysis, and the Imagination*. Redwood City, Stanford University Press.

Chuster, A. (1989) *Um Resgate da Originalidade: os conceitos essenciais da psicanálise em W.R. Bion*. Degraus Cultural, Rio de Janeiro.

Chuster, A. (1995a) Conferência: *"Aspectos históricos, filosóficos e epistemológicos da obra de W.R. Bion,"* III Jornada Científica do Instituto W.R. Bion, Porto Alegre.

Chuster, A. (1995b) *Existe uma escola de Bion?* – III Jornada Científica do Instituto W.R. Bion, Porto Alegre.

Chuster, A. (1995c) *O legado técnico de Bion* – na III Jornada do Instituto W.R. Bion, Porto Alegre.

Chuster, A. (1995d) *O que mudou na prática clínica a partir de Bion?* – III Jornada Científica do Instituto W.R. Bion, Porto Alegre.

Chuster, A. (1996) *Diálogos Psicanalíticos sobre W.R. Bion*. Tipo & Grafia, Rio de Janeiro.

Chuster, A. (1997a) *"The myth of Satan: An Aesthetic View of Bion's Concept of Transformation in O,"* International Centennial Conference on the work of W.R. Bion, Turin, Italy.

Chuster, A. (1997b) *"A influência da Ciência na Obra de W.R. Bion,"* Simpósio Comemorativo *W.R. Bion, 100 anos* organizado pela Sociedade Brasileira de psicanálise do Rio de Janeiro (SBPRJ).

Chuster, A. (1997c) *Cadernos de Bion 1: Seminários com Arnaldo Chuster - Uma teoria do pensar, aprendendo com a experiência.* Organizado por Júlio César Conte, editora Escuta, São Paulo.

Chuster, A. (1997d) A Influência da ciência na psicanálise. *Revista do CEP de Porto Alegre,* ano 6, no 6.

Chuster, A. (1997e) *O Ensino de Bion.* Revista do Instituto Bion, no 1.

Chuster, A. (1997f) *"Facing what can never be reached"* – painel especial sobre *Internet e psicanálise* – International Centennial Conference on the work of W.R. Bion – Turim, Itália.

Chuster, A. (1998) Bion cria de fato uma nova psicanálise? Revista de Psicanálise da SPPA, vol. V, no 3.

Chuster, A. (1999) *W. R. Bion: Novas Leituras, Vol. I: a psicanálise dos modelos científicos aos princípios ético-estéticos.* Companhia de Freud, Rio de Janeiro.

Chuster, A. (2001) Comentários sobre a Conferência de Bion em Paris (1978), Revista da Psicanálise da Sociedade Psicanalítica de Porto Alegre, Volume VIII.

Chuster, A. (2002) *An Oedipal Grid.* Trabalho apresentado na III Conferência Internacional sobre a obra de Bion. Los Angeles, Califórnia.

Chuster, A. (2003) *W.R. Bion: Novas Leituras: a psicanálise dos princípios ético-estéticos à clínica, Companhia de Freud.* Rio de Janeiro.

Chuster, A. (2004) *Os princípios ético-estéticos de observação.* Trabalho apresentado na Conferência Internacional sobre a Obra de Bion, São Paulo.

Chuster, A. (2005a) A Brief Survey in the Difference Between Fantasy and Imagination in the Light of Bion's Ideas. Paper presented to Massachusetts Institute of Psychoanalysis (MIP), Boston, Fevereiro.

Chuster, A. (2005b) Interpretações analíticas e princípios ético-estéticos de observação. Trabalho apresentado, no 44. Congresso da IPA, Rio de Janeiro.

Chuster, A. (2006) *Transformações e Significado* In: *Linguagem e Construção do Pensamento.* Org. Jose Renato Avzaradel, Casa do Psicólogo, São Paulo.

Chuster, A. (2007) As Origens do Inconsciente; arcabouços da mente futura. *Revista da SBP de PA,* vol. XIV, no 2.

Chuster, A. (2009) *Lavorare com Bion nella clínica psicoanalitica.* In Com Bion verso il futuro, editado por Giorgio Corrente, Borla, Roma.

Chuster, A. (2010) The Origins of the Unconscious. In *Primitive Mental States: A Psychoanalytical Exploration of Meaning.* Edited by Jane Van Buren and Shelley Alhanati. Routledge, New York.

Chuster, A. (2011) *O Objeto Psicanalítico.* Edição Instituto W. Bion, Porto Alegre.

Chuster, A. (2012) Cesura e Imaginação Radical: obtendo imagens para a ressignificação da história primitiva no processo analítico. In *Sobre a Linguagem e o Pensar.* Org. Jose Renato Avzaradel. Casa do Psicólogo, São Paulo.

Chuster, A. (2013) *A importância da imaginação do analista na prática clínica: um ensaio sobre a capacidade de se conectar com o mais primitivo.* Trabalho apresentado na X Jornada Científica do Instituto Wilfred Bion, Porto Alegre.

Chuster, A. (2013) *Quando tirar proveito de um mau negócio se torna quase impossível: um ensaio sobre a possessividade e correlatos.* Trabalho apresentado na X Jornada Científica do Instituto Wilfred Bion, Porto Alegre.

Chuster, A. (2013) Bion: Uma leitura Complexa na contemporaneidade. Curso apresentado no XXIV Congresso Brasileiro de Psicanálise, Campo Grande, Mato Grosso do Sul.

Chuster, A. (2014) *A Lonesome Road: Essays on the Complexity of W.R. Bion's Work.* TrioStudios/Karnac, Rio de Janeiro.

Chuster, A. (2015) *A Personalidade Irascível,* Reverie: Revista da Soc. Psicanalítica de Fortaleza, vol. 8.

Chuster, A. (2016) *Em uma sessão estou interessado naquilo que não sei*. Trabalho apresentado na IX Jornada de Psicanálise: Bion 2016, organizado pela Sociedade Brasileira de Psicanálise de São Paulo.

Chuster, A. (2017a) *Experiences with Wild Thoughts*. Inédito.

Chuster, A. (2017b) Comentários ao Trabalho: *O Desamparo e a Mente do Analista* de Leda Spessoto. Sociedade Brasileira de Psicanálise de São Paulo.

Chuster, A. (2017c) *Comentários ao trabalho de Altamirando Mattos de Oliveira Filho*. Sociedade Brasileira de Psicanálise do Rio de Janeiro.

Chuster, A. (2018a) *Simetria e Objeto Psicanalítico; desafiando paradigmas com W.R. Bion*. Trio Studio, Rio de Janeiro.

Chuster, A. (2018b) Serendipidade e Memória do Futuro: pensamentos selvagens em busca de uma descoberta. Trabalho apresentado na Jornada Bion da SBPSP, São Paulo.

Chuster, A. (2018c) *Capacidade negativa; um caminho em busca da luz*. Inédito.

Chuster, A. (2018d) *Sortilégio*. Trabalho apresentado na Jornada Bion da SBPSP, São Paulo.

Chuster, A. (2023) *Language of Psychoanalytical Range, Bion's Transcendental Difference*. Hedges Publishers, Los Angeles.

Chuster, A., Soares, G., & Trachtenberg, R. (2014) *A Obra Complexa*. Editora Sulina, Porto Alegre.

Chuster, A. & Trachtenberg, R. (2009) *As Sete Invejas Capitais*. Artmed, Porto Alegre.

Meltzer, D. (1996) *Meltzer em São Paulo: seminários clínicos*. Casa do Psicólogo, São Paulo.

Laplanche, J. (1989) *New Foundations for Psychoanalysis* (D. Macey, Trans.). Basil Blackwell. (Original work published 1987).

Index

Note: Page numbers in *italics* represent figures; and those followed by "n" refer to notes.